The Cortisol Detox Diet Plan

28 Days to Reset Stress Hormones, Burn Belly Fat, Boost Energy, and Restore Calm Naturally

Abigail Douglas

Table of Contents

The Cortisol Detox Diet Plan 1

How to Use This Book 20

Preface 22

Introduction 29

PART I — THE SCIENCE OF STRESS AND CORTISOL RESET 36

Chapter 1 37

Understanding Cortisol — The Hidden Hormone Behind Stress and Weight Gain 37

What Cortisol Really Does in the Body 37

Healthy Stress vs. Chronic Stress 39

The Cortisol–Weight Connection............................ 40

Why Caffeine, Sugar, and Sleep Deprivation Worsen Cortisol Overload... 42

The Hidden Cost of Always Being "On".................... 43

Chapter 2 46

Signs Your Cortisol Is Out of Balance....................... 46

Physical Signs: When Your Body Starts Whispering 47

Emotional Signs: When Calm Feels Out of Reach 49

Biological Markers — and When to Seek Medical Advice 50

How Modern Life Keeps Cortisol Stuck on High 52

The Turning Point 53

Chapter 3 56

How Diet Affects Stress Hormones 56

The Link Between Blood Sugar and Cortisol 56

Anti-Inflammatory vs. Pro-Inflammatory Foods 58

Why Skipping Meals Increases Cortisol Spikes 60

Foods Rich in Magnesium, Omega-3s, and Adaptogenic Nutrients 62

The Way You Eat Matters As Much as What You Eat 65

Chapter 4 67

The Science of Reset — Preparing for Your 28-Day Cortisol Detox 67

How the Detox Plan Works (Science-Backed, Not Restrictive) 68

Preparing Your Kitchen: What to Remove and What to Stock 69

Morning, Afternoon, and Evening Rituals That Stabilize Cortisol 72

Gentle Introduction to Hydration, Herbal Teas, and Deep Breathing 75

    Hydration: The Forgotten Detox 76

    Herbal Teas: Nature's Calm in a Cup 76

    Deep Breathing: The Body's Built-in Reset 77

The Art of Beginning Again 78

PART II — THE 28-DAY CORTISOL DETOX PLAN 80

Chapter 5 81

Week 1 — Calm the Chaos: Restoring Inner Balance 81

The Purpose of Week One 82

Your 7-Day Meal Rhythm 82

Key Foods for Week One 85

Stress Relief Rituals for This Week 87

A Gentle Reminder 89

Chapter 6 92

Week 2 — Nourish to Heal: Rebuilding the Gut and Adrenals 92

Why Gut and Adrenal Healing Go Hand in Hand . 93

The Focus of Week Two: Nourishment as Medicine . 94

Gut-Friendly Meals: Bone Broth, Fermented Foods, and Leafy Greens 95

Morning Smoothies with Adaptogens 97

Mindful Breathing and Self-Care Habits 99

A Deeper Truth About Healing 101

Chapter 7 103

Week 3 — Revitalize Energy: From Burnout to Brilliance 103

The Focus of Week 3 104

Energizing Breakfasts: High-Protein, Slow-Carb Fuel

.... 105

1. Savory Protein Bowl 106

2. Greek Yogurt Parfait with Slow Carbs............. 106

3. Warm Cinnamon Oats with Almond Butter..... 107

4. Power Smoothie 108

Movement for Vitality: Yoga, Walking & Stretching 108

1. Yoga: Move with Breath 109

2. Walking: The Most Underrated Energy Medicine 110

3. Stretching: Flexibility for the Nervous System 110

Resetting the Sleep Cycle with Natural Cues 111

1. Morning Sunlight Exposure 112

2. Evening Wind-Down Ritual 113

3. Cool, Quiet, Comfort-Promoting Bedroom 113

4. The 10–3–2–1–0 Rule (Modified for Stress Recovery) 114

The Beauty of Week 3 115

Chapter 8 117

Week 4 — Sustain and Strengthen: Living Stress-Free Beyond Detox 117

The Focus of Week 4 118

Reintroducing Occasional Treats Without Triggering Cortisol 118

How to Reintroduce Treats Safely 119

Managing Deadlines, Relationships, and Emotions Mindfully 120

Turning Daily Routines Into Wellness Rituals 122

Your New Relationship With Stress 123

Beyond the 28 Days 124

PART III — RECIPES & RITUALS FOR HORMONAL BALANCE 126

Chapter 9 127

Cortisol-Lowering Recipes for Every Meal 127

Breakfasts to Steady Blood Sugar 128

Nourishing Lunches That Fuel Calm 130

Soothing Dinners for Better Sleep 131

Herbal Teas, Snacks, and Smoothies 133

    Herbal Teas for Calm 133

    Low-Stress Snacks 134

    Adaptogenic Smoothies 135

Your Cortisol-Calming Weekly Recipe Rotation..... 135

    Monday – Reset & Ground 136

    Tuesday – Digest & Restore 137

    Wednesday – Energize Gently 138

    Thursday – Balance & Focus................................ 139

    Friday – Support & Soothe 140

    Saturday – Nourish & Enjoy................................. 141

Sunday – Reset & Prepare 142

How to Use This Rotation for the Entire Detox 142

How to Use This Chapter Long-Term 144

A Final Note on Food and Freedom 144

Chapter 10 146

Stress Detox Rituals and Lifestyle Blueprint 146

Breathing Patterns That Reduce Cortisol in 60 Seconds 146

Journaling, Gratitude, and Emotional Regulation 148

Gratitude as a Biological Tool 149

Emotional Regulation: Responding Instead of Reacting 149

Creating Your Daily "Calm Schedule" 150

    Morning Anchor 151

    Midday Anchor 151

    Evening Anchor 152

Nature Therapy, Grounding, and Mindfulness 152

Your Long-Term Lifestyle Blueprint 154

A Final Reflection 155

PART IV — LONG-TERM SUCCESS AND SELF-MASTERY 157

Chapter 11 158

Rebalancing for Life — Your Post-Detox Maintenance Plan 158

The 80/20 Rule: Flexibility Without Fear 159

How to Use the 80/20 Rule in Practice 159

Recognizing Early Signs of Cortisol Flare-Ups .. 160

Your Cortisol Recovery Toolkit 161

Adapting the Plan During Travel, Work Stress, or Life Changes 163

The Truth About Long-Term Balance 164

Your New Relationship With Your Body 165

Chapter 12 167

The 7-Day Emergency Stress Reset 167

How This Reset Works 168

The Core Rules (Keep These Simple) 169

Day 1: Stop the Bleeding 169

Day 2: Ground the Body 170

Day 3: Calm the Nervous System 171

Day 4: Restore Energy Gently 172

Day 5: Release Emotional Load 173

Day 6: Rebuild Rhythm 174

Day 7: Reset Forward 174

Emergency Reset Shortcuts (When You're Very Overwhelmed)... 175

What This Reset Is (and Isn't) 176

A Final Word 177

Chapter 13 178

Mind Over Cortisol — The Psychology of Lasting Calm 178

The Thought–Stress Connection 178

Rewiring Your Brain's Reaction to Triggers 179

Building Emotional Resilience and Inner Peace .. 181

Living With Awareness and Lightness 182

Conclusion — A New Rhythm of Living 183

Acknowledgment 186

Copyright © 2025 by Abigail Douglas

All rights reserved. No part of this book may be copied, reproduced, stored, or transmitted in any form or by any means—electronic, mechanical, photocopying, recording, or otherwise without prior written permission from the publisher, except for brief quotations used in reviews or scholarly works.

Disclaimer

The information in this book is provided for educational and informational purposes only and is not intended as a substitute for professional medical advice, diagnosis, or treatment.

Always seek the advice of your physician, qualified health provider, or registered dietitian with any questions you may have regarding a medical condition, dietary change, or wellness practice.

Never disregard professional medical advice or delay seeking it because of something you have read in this book.

The author and publisher disclaim any liability for any loss or damage arising directly or indirectly from the use of this material.

Every effort has been made to ensure the accuracy of information presented; however, individual results will vary, and readers are encouraged to honor their unique health needs.

How to Use This Book

This book is meant to be lived, not merely read.

Each section has been designed to meet you where you are — whether you're just beginning to understand your body's stress response or you're ready to commit to a full 28-day reset.

Start with **Part I** to learn how cortisol shapes your energy, sleep, and weight.

Move into **Part II**, the **28-Day Cortisol Detox Plan**, where daily guidance, recipes, and rituals help you rebuild balance step by step.

In **Part III**, explore nourishing recipes and calming practices you can return to long after the detox is complete.

Finally, **Part IV** will show you how to sustain your new rhythm for life — turning calm into your daily default.

Keep a journal nearby. Highlight what resonates. Adapt

the meals and rituals to your taste and schedule.

Above all, listen to your body — it speaks the language of balance when we slow down enough to hear it.

Preface

Why This Book Exists

Stress has quietly become one of the most underestimated health disruptors of our time.

Not the obvious kind—the occasional hard day or short-term pressure—but the chronic, low-grade stress that settles into daily life and never quite leaves. The kind that shows up as stubborn belly fat, constant fatigue, poor sleep, anxiety, cravings, hormonal imbalance, brain fog, and a body that feels perpetually out of sync.

For many people, the missing piece behind these struggles isn't a lack of discipline or motivation.

It's **cortisol**.

Cortisol is often called the stress hormone, but that label barely scratches the surface. Cortisol regulates blood sugar, energy levels, inflammation, sleep cycles, mood, and fat storage. When it's balanced, the body feels resilient and calm. When it's chronically elevated—or poorly regulated—it can quietly sabotage weight loss, digestion, sleep, and emotional well-being.

This book exists because too many people are trying to heal stress-related symptoms with strategies that unintentionally make cortisol worse: extreme dieting, skipping meals, over-exercising, constant caffeine, rigid routines, and self-criticism disguised as "discipline."

This is not another weight-loss plan.

Not another restrictive detox.

Not another promise of quick fixes.

This is a **cortisol detox diet plan** designed for real life—one that focuses on hormonal balance, nervous system regulation, sustainable weight management, and long-term calm.

A Different Kind of Detox

When most people hear detox, they think of deprivation.

Juices instead of meals.

Rules instead of rhythm.

Short-term results followed by burnout.

This book takes a completely different approach.

The **28-day cortisol reset outlined** here is science-aligned, nourishment-focused, and intentionally gentle. Instead of forcing the body into compliance, it teaches the body safety—because safety is what allows cortisol levels to normalize naturally.

You'll learn how:

- Blood sugar stability directly affects cortisol and belly fat
- Certain foods calm stress hormones instead of triggering them
- Simple daily rituals can lower cortisol in minutes

- Sleep, light exposure, and timing matter more than willpower
- Emotional regulation and mindset are essential for lasting calm

This is a **stress detox plan** that works with your biology—not against it.

Why Diet Alone Isn't Enough

Cortisol imbalance doesn't begin in the kitchen alone.

It begins in thought patterns, emotional load, sleep deprivation, overstimulation, and the constant pressure to perform.

That's why this book goes beyond food.

Alongside cortisol-lowering meals, you'll find:

- Stress-reducing breathing techniques
- Gut-healing nutrition strategies
- Adrenal support through lifestyle rhythm

- Mind-body practices for emotional balance
- A psychology-based approach to lasting calm

This is a **holistic cortisol detox**—one that addresses weight, energy, mood, and mental clarity together.

Who This Book Is For

This book is for anyone who feels like stress has become the background noise of their life.

It's for those who:

- Feel tired even after sleeping
- Struggle with stress-related weight gain or belly fat
- Experience anxiety, irritability, or burnout
- Crave sugar, caffeine, or constant stimulation
- Want a natural way to balance hormones and restore energy

You don't need a diagnosis.

You don't need perfection.

You don't need to "fix" yourself.

You need understanding—and a plan that respects your nervous system.

What You'll Gain

By the end of this book, you won't just know how to lower cortisol.

You'll know how to live in a way that prevents it from spiraling again.

You'll have:

- A repeatable cortisol detox meal framework
- A weekly recipe rotation for calm and energy
- A stress-reset toolkit for high-pressure days
- A post-detox maintenance plan
- A mindset shift that replaces urgency with ease

Most importantly, you'll walk away with something far more valuable than a diet:

A **new rhythm of living**—one where nourishment replaces stress, balance replaces burnout, and calm becomes your default state, not a rare achievement.

This book isn't about doing more.

It's about doing *what actually works*.

And it begins with understanding cortisol—not as something to fight, but as something to guide back into balance.

Welcome to the reset.

Introduction

When Stress Becomes the Body's Language

If you're holding this book, chances are your body has been trying to tell you something.

Maybe it started quietly—with fatigue that sleep no longer fixes, weight that seems to cling no matter what you eat, a mind that won't slow down even when life finally does. Or maybe it arrived louder—through anxiety, burnout, stubborn belly fat, restless nights, cravings, or a constant feeling of being "on edge."

What many people don't realize is that these experiences are often connected by one powerful, misunderstood hormone: **cortisol**.

Cortisol is not your enemy. It was designed to protect you. It helps you wake up in the morning, respond to challenges, and survive moments of danger. But when modern life keeps that survival switch turned on—through constant pressure, poor sleep, blood sugar swings, emotional overload, and endless stimulation—cortisol stops being helpful. It becomes exhausting.

This book exists because stress today isn't rare or temporary. It's chronic. And the body always adapts—sometimes in ways that leave us feeling confused, frustrated, or disconnected from ourselves.

This is not another diet that asks you to push harder.

It's not a detox that demands restriction, punishment, or perfection.

And it's not a promise to "fix" you—because you were never broken.

This is a **reset**.

A return to rhythm.

A return to nourishment.

A return to listening.

What This Book Is Really About

At its core, this book is about **safety**.

When your body feels safe, cortisol settles.

When cortisol settles, weight becomes easier to manage.

Energy begins to return.

Sleep deepens.

Cravings soften.

The mind clears.

And calm stops feeling like something you have to chase.

Through the chapters ahead, you'll learn how stress hormones actually work—and more importantly, how everyday choices quietly influence them. You'll discover why certain foods calm the nervous system while others keep it on high alert. You'll understand how sleep, light, movement, breath, emotions, and even thoughts shape your hormonal environment.

Most importantly, you'll be guided through a **gentle, science-aligned 28-day cortisol reset**—not to overhaul your life, but to teach your body how to come back into balance naturally.

What Makes This Approach Different

This plan doesn't believe in extremes.

It doesn't rely on willpower.

And it doesn't ask you to disconnect from real life.

Instead, it works with:

- Balanced meals that stabilize blood sugar instead of stressing it
- Simple rituals that calm the nervous system in minutes
- Mindset shifts that reduce stress at its source
- Movement and rest that restore energy without depletion

- Psychological tools that help you respond to life instead of bracing against it

You'll move through four weeks of progressive support—calming chaos, healing digestion and adrenals, restoring energy, and learning how to sustain balance long after the reset ends.

And because life doesn't pause after a program, you'll also find:

- A post-detox maintenance plan
- An emergency 7-day stress reset
- A lifestyle blueprint for real-world challenges
- Tools for emotional resilience and mental calm

This book doesn't just help you lower cortisol.

It helps you understand yourself.

Who This Book Is For

This book is for anyone who feels like their body is

carrying more than it should.

For the woman who's tired of feeling wired but exhausted.

For the person who eats "right" but still feels off.

For those navigating busy lives, emotional seasons, work pressure, caregiving, or constant mental load.

For anyone who senses that stress—not lack of discipline—is at the root of their struggle.

You don't need a diagnosis to begin.

You don't need perfect habits.

You don't need to start over.

You just need a willingness to slow down enough to listen.

A Gentle Invitation

As you read, move at your own pace.

There is no race here.

No finish line to prove yourself at.

Let this book be a companion, not a command.

A guide, not a judge.

Because the truth is simple—and quietly powerful:

Your body knows how to heal.

It just needs the right conditions.

This book will help you create them.

And what follows isn't just a detox.

It's the beginning of a calmer, steadier, more sustainable way of living—one where nourishment replaces urgency, balance replaces burnout, and stress no longer runs the show.

Let's begin.

PART I — THE SCIENCE OF STRESS AND CORTISOL RESET

Chapter 1

Understanding Cortisol — The Hidden Hormone Behind Stress and Weight Gain

It usually begins quietly — a few late nights, a bit of extra caffeine, a skipped breakfast here and there. You tell yourself you're just tired. Then, somewhere between exhaustion and restlessness, your body starts whispering that something is off: stubborn belly fat that wasn't there before, cravings that ignore logic, a mind that won't slow down even when the lights are off.

What you're feeling is not weakness. It's your body's alarm system — and cortisol is the messenger ringing the bell.

What Cortisol Really Does in the

Body

Cortisol is often painted as the "bad guy," but in truth, it's one of the most intelligent hormones you possess. Produced by your adrenal glands — two small, triangular powerhouses that rest above your kidneys — cortisol is designed to help you **survive**.

When you wake up in the morning, cortisol rises naturally to shake you out of sleep, sharpen your focus, and raise your blood sugar just enough to fuel movement and thought.

When a deadline looms or danger appears, cortisol steps in again, mobilizing stored energy so you can think fast and act quickly.

In moderation, cortisol is your ally — a steady hand that keeps you alert, balanced, and capable of responding to life's challenges. The problem begins when the alarm never turns off.

When chronic stress keeps your system on high alert — whether from overwork, worry, poor sleep, or emotional strain — cortisol production stays elevated far longer than it was ever meant to. The hormone that once kept you safe begins to wear you down from within: disrupting digestion, dulling immunity, and telling your body to hold on to every calorie as if famine were around the corner.

Healthy Stress vs. Chronic Stress

Not all stress is harmful. **Healthy stress**, or "eustress," is the temporary kind that pushes you toward growth — the mild tension before a big presentation, the surge of energy during a workout, the excitement of learning something new. Once the challenge passes, cortisol levels naturally drop, returning your body to calm equilibrium.

Chronic stress, on the other hand, is the slow leak you don't notice until it floods your system. It's the kind that never ends — unanswered emails, financial worry, constant multitasking, unresolved emotions. Your body interprets every one of these as potential danger.

When stress becomes your baseline, cortisol becomes your background music — constant, humming, and exhausting. Sleep loses its depth, cravings intensify, and even your best dietary choices can't undo the message your hormones are sending: *store fat, just in case.*

The Cortisol–Weight Connection

Few things frustrate people more than doing "everything right" — eating well, exercising — and still watching the scale refuse to move. The missing link is often **cortisol**.

When cortisol levels stay elevated, several key changes occur:

- **Insulin resistance increases.** Your cells stop responding efficiently to insulin, causing blood sugar to linger in your bloodstream and eventually be stored as fat — particularly around the abdomen.
- **Appetite hormones misfire.** Leptin, the hormone that signals fullness, becomes blunted. Ghrelin, which triggers hunger, rises. The result: you feel hungry even when you've eaten enough.
- **Muscle breaks down for fuel.** Your body begins converting muscle tissue into glucose to sustain prolonged "alert mode," which further lowers metabolism.
- **Fat prefers the midsection.** Visceral fat — the kind that pads your organs — produces its own cortisol, trapping you in a self-perpetuating loop of stress and storage.

It's not vanity weight; it's biological armor. Your body believes you're under threat, so it prepares you to survive rather than thrive.

Why Caffeine, Sugar, and Sleep Deprivation Worsen Cortisol Overload

In a culture that glorifies busyness, three common habits silently fuel cortisol chaos:

1. Caffeine:

That morning cup (or three) of coffee triggers the same adrenal response as a mild stressor. When consumed in excess or too late in the day, caffeine keeps cortisol elevated long after you need it. Over time, the adrenal glands fatigue, leaving you wired yet depleted — jittery in the day, restless at night.

2. Sugar:

Refined sugar causes rapid spikes and crashes in blood

glucose. Each crash prompts a cortisol surge to stabilize energy levels, keeping the stress loop active. Pair sugar with caffeine, and your body rides a hormonal rollercoaster that ends in cravings and exhaustion.

3. Sleep Deprivation:

Lack of deep, restorative sleep disrupts the natural circadian rhythm that governs cortisol release. Instead of peaking in the morning and tapering at night, cortisol stays elevated around the clock, making it harder to fall asleep — and harder still to burn fat.

Chronic poor sleep is one of the fastest ways to convince your body that danger never ends.

The Hidden Cost of Always Being "On"

We've learned to mistake stimulation for productivity. The glow of a phone at midnight feels like control. The extra hour of work feels like progress. But biologically, it's confusion.

Your body doesn't recognize "work email" versus "wild predator." It only registers tension, noise, and urgency — and it responds the same way it has for millennia: with cortisol.

Learning to regulate this hormone begins not with punishment or deprivation, but with awareness. Once you understand that your stress response is ancient, intelligent, and protective, you can begin to work with it — not against it.

The chapters that follow will show you how food, rest, movement, and mindful living can re-teach your body what safety feels like. Because when your body feels safe, it stops hoarding energy and starts releasing it. That's when healing — and sustainable weight loss — finally begins.

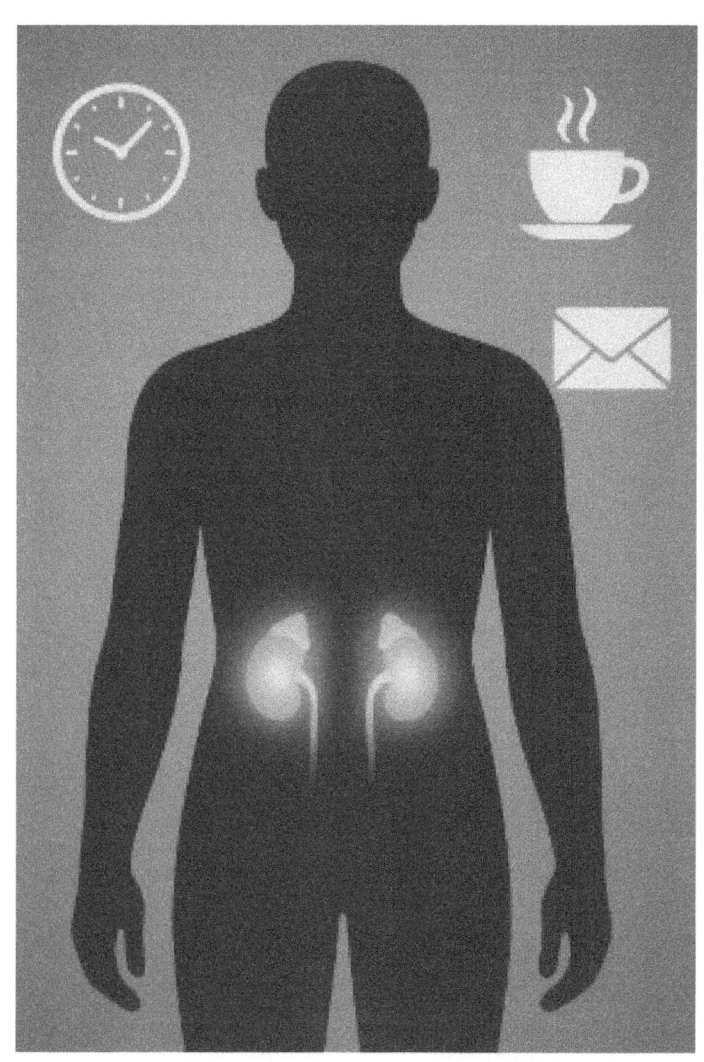

Chapter 2

Signs Your Cortisol Is Out of Balance

You can't always see stress — but your body feels it long before your mind admits it. It shows up quietly at first: a little extra weight around your middle, a short fuse with people you love, the sense that rest never feels like enough. Many of us call this "just getting older" or "being busy," but underneath the surface, your hormones are trying to tell you something.

Cortisol, the hormone that keeps you alert and steady, becomes disruptive when it stops cycling in rhythm. Instead of rising with the morning sun and falling at night, it begins to leak through the cracks of your day, showing up when you're supposed to rest and disappearing when you need energy most.

Recognizing its signals early is the first step toward

reclaiming calm, energy, and emotional steadiness.

Physical Signs: When Your Body Starts Whispering

1. Stubborn Belly Fat

If you've noticed weight settling around your waistline despite eating well or exercising, it may not be about calories at all — it's cortisol chemistry.

When stress hormones surge, the body redirects fat storage to the abdomen, near vital organs. This type of fat, called visceral fat, produces its own cortisol, locking you into a self-feeding loop. It's your body's attempt to protect you from a threat that never ends.

2. Persistent Fatigue

Waking up exhausted, craving coffee before conversation, or feeling like every task demands triple effort — these are not personality traits. They're adrenal distress signals. Chronic stress dulls the adrenal glands' ability to release cortisol at the right time, leaving you drained when you should feel alert.

3. Poor Sleep

When cortisol stays high into the evening, it tells the body that night is not a safe time to rest. You may fall asleep only to wake at 2 a.m. with racing thoughts or a pounding heart. Over time, the cycle reverses entirely: low cortisol in the morning (no energy) and high cortisol at night (no sleep).

4. Weakened Immunity and Slow Recovery

Frequent colds, prolonged healing, and muscle soreness that lingers longer than it should are subtle consequences of cortisol excess. Your immune system, once sharp and responsive, becomes sluggish under chronic stress.

5. Digestive Distress

Bloating, indigestion, or alternating constipation and urgency can arise because cortisol diverts blood flow away from digestion toward "fight or flight." Even the healthiest meals lose their benefit when eaten in a stressed state.

Emotional Signs: When Calm Feels Out of Reach

Hormones don't just regulate metabolism — they influence mood, motivation, and perspective. When cortisol is mismanaged, emotions begin to swing.

1. Irritability and Mood Swings

One minute you're fine; the next, even small frustrations feel enormous. That volatility is biochemical, not moral failure. Elevated cortisol depletes serotonin and dopamine, the neurotransmitters that keep your emotional balance steady.

2. Anxiety and Uneasy Restlessness

Chronic high cortisol keeps your nervous system locked in alert mode. Your heart rate stays slightly elevated; your breathing shallow. You feel edgy even when life seems calm. Over time, anxiety becomes your default frequency.

3. Burnout and Emotional Numbness

At the far end of the stress spectrum lies burnout — the stage where your system can no longer produce sufficient cortisol. You don't feel anxious anymore; you feel nothing. Joy, creativity, and passion flatten out. This is adrenal depletion, the body's final attempt to protect itself from collapse.

Biological Markers — and When to Seek Medical Advice

While most symptoms can be observed intuitively, sometimes laboratory testing provides clarity.

- **Cortisol rhythm testing** (saliva or blood) can reveal if levels spike or crash at the wrong times.
- **Blood sugar patterns** may show instability even in non-diabetic individuals.
- **Thyroid panels** sometimes appear "off" because chronic stress suppresses thyroid function.
- **High blood pressure or elevated triglycerides** can also point to cortisol excess.

If you experience continuous fatigue, unexplained weight gain around the midsection, or insomnia that lasts longer than a few weeks, consult your physician or an endocrinologist. Functional-medicine practitioners can also help interpret results that fall within the "normal" range but are sub-optimal for you.

Seeking professional help isn't weakness — it's strategy. Early awareness prevents long-term damage to the adrenal-thyroid axis and overall metabolic health.

How Modern Life Keeps Cortisol Stuck on High

Our ancestors' stress lasted minutes. Ours lasts months — and it hides in plain sight.

1. Blue Light Overexposure

Screens trick your brain into thinking it's midday even at midnight. Blue light delays melatonin release, keeps cortisol elevated, and erases the body's sense of time. That glow in your palm is a miniature sunrise disrupting every hormonal rhythm you have.

2. Overworking and Constant Availability

Digital culture rewards exhaustion disguised as productivity. "Just one more email" becomes a 16-hour cortisol drip. The human nervous system was never meant to process dozens of notifications an hour; each one triggers a micro-burst of adrenaline and cortisol.

3. Unstable Eating Patterns

Skipping meals, surviving on caffeine, or eating late into the night confuses your metabolic clock. When blood sugar dips, cortisol surges to bring it back up — another unnecessary alarm your body must extinguish.

4. Emotional Overload and Information Fatigue

Even when your body sits still, your mind may be sprinting through an endless feed of comparisons, crises, and headlines. Emotional stress is processed as physical stress; your adrenals don't differentiate between a looming deadline and a painful news cycle.

The Turning Point

The truth is simple: your body is not broken — it's adaptive. Every symptom you feel is an intelligent response to an environment that has forgotten how to rest. Cortisol imbalance isn't a verdict; it's a message. Once you learn to listen — to the tiredness behind your morning coffee, the irritability behind your overthinking, the craving behind your fatigue — you gain the power to change it.

The next chapters will guide you through how to calm that internal alarm.

You'll discover what foods, habits, and rhythms teach the body safety again — so that cortisol can return to its natural flow: high in the morning to spark your day, low at night to cradle you into deep, restorative sleep.

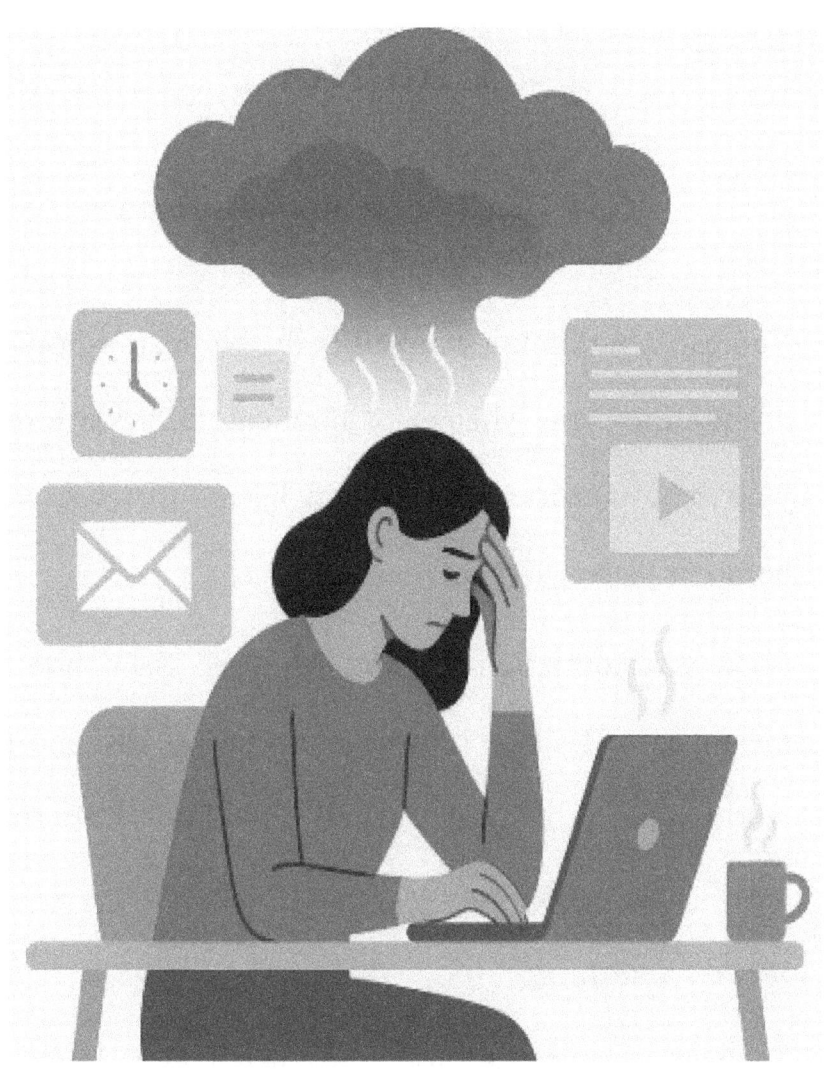

Chapter 3

How Diet Affects Stress Hormones

You can't outthink a stressed body. No matter how many affirmations you whisper or how carefully you organize your day, your nervous system listens to what you eat before it listens to what you say.

Food is information — not just fuel. Each bite sends messages that shape how your hormones respond to the world. The right meal can tell your body, *"You're safe now."* The wrong one whispers, *"Something's wrong — stay on guard."*

To heal from stress, you must teach your body peace through nourishment.

The Link Between Blood Sugar and

Cortisol

Cortisol and blood sugar are dance partners — and when one trips, the other falls.

Your body depends on stable blood sugar to maintain energy and focus. When you go too long without eating or when your meal is mostly refined carbs or sugar, your blood sugar spikes and then crashes. In that crash, your body panics. It releases cortisol to pull stored glucose into your bloodstream, ensuring your brain still gets fuel.

At first, this survival mechanism works beautifully. But when it happens multiple times a day — from skipped breakfasts, sugary snacks, or late-night eating — cortisol stays elevated far longer than intended.

Your body begins to interpret your daily diet as a series of emergencies.

Over time, these constant fluctuations can lead to:

- Fatigue and brain fog from erratic energy levels
- Cravings for sugar or caffeine as quick fixes
- Weight gain, especially around the midsection
- Irritability or "hangry" moods that feel beyond your control

Every unsteady meal becomes a mini stress signal. And each balanced meal becomes a message of calm.

To stabilize this relationship, **pair protein, healthy fat, and fiber** at every meal. A breakfast of eggs, avocado, and leafy greens sends a different message to your adrenal glands than a cup of coffee and a muffin. It says, *"We're nourished, not starving."*

Balanced blood sugar is the foundation of emotional stability.

Anti-Inflammatory vs. Pro-Inflammatory Foods

Chronic inflammation is the quiet accomplice of high

cortisol. When your body is inflamed, it produces more stress hormones; when cortisol is high, it promotes inflammation — a biochemical loop that burns through energy, mood, and health.

Pro-inflammatory foods — processed sugars, refined oils (like soybean, corn, or canola), white flour, and trans fats — keep the stress response simmering. They inflame the gut, disrupt digestion, and impair nutrient absorption. Each processed snack you eat might satisfy for a moment but leaves behind microscopic damage that signals your body to stay in fight mode.

Anti-inflammatory foods, in contrast, quiet the immune system and reduce cortisol naturally. Think of them as internal healers:

- **Leafy greens** like spinach, kale, and arugula — rich in chlorophyll and magnesium

- **Fatty fish** like salmon and sardines — sources of omega-3s that regulate inflammation
- **Colorful fruits and vegetables** — packed with antioxidants that repair cellular stress
- **Nuts, seeds, and olive oil** — nourishing fats that soothe the nervous system

Each of these foods acts like a peace treaty within your body, calming internal conflict. They don't just fill your stomach — they rebuild balance.

Why Skipping Meals Increases Cortisol Spikes

Skipping meals is one of the fastest ways to trigger cortisol surges, yet it's one of the most common habits in modern life. You rush through the morning, powered by caffeine. Lunch becomes optional. Dinner arrives too late — and suddenly, your hunger feels primal.

Here's what happens behind the scenes:

When you skip meals, blood sugar drops. Your body interprets that drop as an emergency and releases cortisol to raise glucose levels by breaking down muscle tissue into usable energy. It's a brilliant short-term response — but destructive when repeated daily.

This pattern leads to:

- **Muscle loss** and slower metabolism
- **Fat storage**, especially visceral fat
- **Sugar and carb cravings**, as your brain seeks fast energy
- **Irritability and mood crashes**, as cortisol and blood sugar collide

Your body doesn't understand "dieting." It only understands feast or famine. Skipping meals feels like famine — and cortisol rises to protect you. Ironically, this protection mechanism blocks fat loss and exhausts your adrenal system.

The solution is rhythm, not restriction.

Eat within an hour of waking, and avoid going more than 4–5 hours between meals. Think of your body like a fire: steady logs (protein and fats) burn slowly, while twigs (sugar and refined carbs) burn fast and leave ashes. Keep the fire consistent, and your hormones will stay warm but calm.

Foods Rich in Magnesium, Omega-3s, and Adaptogenic Nutrients

If cortisol is the spark, nutrients are the water that cools the flame. Certain nutrients act like biochemical tranquilizers — not sedating, but steadying. They support your adrenal glands, regulate blood pressure, and promote a calm, focused mood.

1. Magnesium: The Calming Mineral

Magnesium helps deactivate adrenaline once a stress event

has passed. It regulates blood sugar, relaxes muscles, and helps your nervous system switch from "fight or flight" to "rest and digest."

Low magnesium levels are linked to anxiety, insomnia, and heightened stress reactivity.

Sources: spinach, pumpkin seeds, almonds, dark chocolate (in moderation), and avocado.

A small magnesium-rich snack before bed can even help smooth the night's cortisol curve, improving sleep depth and morning energy.

2. Omega-3 Fatty Acids: The Hormone Harmonizers

Omega-3s act as messengers that lower inflammation and stabilize mood hormones like serotonin and dopamine.

They help reduce the body's overproduction of cortisol during stress and support brain function.

Sources: salmon, sardines, flaxseeds, chia seeds, walnuts, and algae oil.

Omega-3s not only heal the body but sharpen emotional resilience — reducing reactivity and grounding mood swings.

3. Adaptogenic Nutrients and Herbs

Adaptogens are nature's stress balancers — plants that help your body adapt to physical or emotional strain without overstimulating it. They nourish the adrenal glands, improve energy, and promote endurance.

Common adaptogens:

- **Ashwagandha** – reduces cortisol and anxiety, enhances restfulness
- **Rhodiola rosea** – supports focus and endurance during fatigue
- **Holy basil (Tulsi)** – balances blood sugar and emotional stress
- **Licorice root** – supports adrenal recovery in exhaustion (use moderately under guidance)

Including small doses of adaptogens in teas, smoothies, or morning tonics can gradually retrain your stress response.

The Way You Eat Matters As Much as What You Eat

Even the healthiest meal can become stressful if eaten hurriedly. Cortisol spikes when you eat in fight-or-flight mode because digestion shuts down when the body perceives danger.

Before every meal, pause for ten seconds. Breathe deeply. Let your nervous system know that you are safe enough to digest.

That single breath changes how your body receives your food.

In the end, the cortisol-detox diet isn't about perfection — it's about peace.

Peace on your plate. Peace in your bloodstream. Peace in your breath.

Every balanced bite is a whisper to your body: *You can relax now. We have enough.*

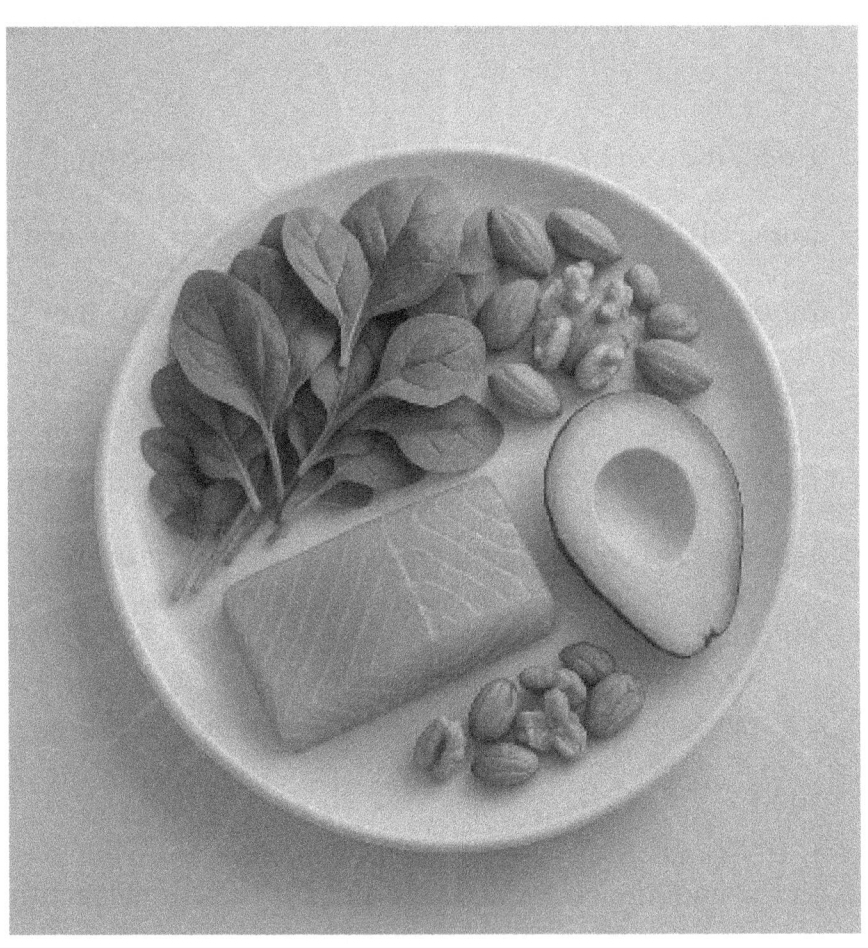

Chapter 4

The Science of Reset — Preparing for Your 28-Day Cortisol Detox

There comes a moment in every healing journey when awareness turns into action — when knowledge stops being a concept and becomes a lifestyle.

That moment begins here.

By now, you understand cortisol not as an enemy but as a messenger — a hormone that only shouts when your body's balance has gone unheard. The goal of the **28-Day Cortisol Detox** isn't to "fight" your hormones or starve your stress away. It's to help your body remember what safety feels like.

This plan is not about restriction; it's about rhythm. You'll feed, hydrate, and rest your body in ways that reprogram your stress response — gently, naturally, and sustainably.

Every habit you form in these four weeks teaches your brain and adrenals a new language: peace is possible.

How the Detox Plan Works (Science-Backed, Not Restrictive)

When people hear the word detox, they often imagine deprivation — green juices, hunger pangs, and endless rules. This is not that.

The **Cortisol Detox Plan** is grounded in **science and nourishment**, not starvation. It works by addressing the four pillars that govern stress and hormonal health:

1. **Blood Sugar Regulation** — Stabilizing glucose prevents cortisol spikes and crashes throughout the day. You'll do this through balanced meals, mindful eating, and eliminating inflammatory sugar cycles.

2. **Inflammation Reduction** — Every anti-inflammatory meal calms your immune system, signaling your adrenals that you're not under attack.

3. **Nervous System Recalibration** — Through gentle movement, deep breathing, and rest, your body learns to leave fight-or-flight mode.

4. **Restorative Nutrition & Hydration** — Adaptogenic herbs, minerals, and hydration habits repair adrenal function and rebuild your energy reserves.

You're not cleansing your body from toxins — you're re-teaching it harmony.

Over the next 28 days, you'll shift from survival to restoration — meal by meal, breath by breath, choice by choice.

Preparing Your Kitchen: What to Remove and What

to Stock

Think of your kitchen as your control center. Every ingredient you bring in can either calm or confuse your hormones. This reset begins by curating an environment that supports the biology of peace.

What to Remove: The Cortisol Agitators

Start by clearing out foods that keep your body in a stress loop:

- **Refined sugars** and sweetened snacks — they spike insulin and cortisol simultaneously.
- **Highly processed foods** with artificial additives, flavor enhancers, and trans fats.
- **Refined carbohydrates** like white bread, pasta, and pastries.
- **Excess caffeine and alcohol** — they jolt your adrenals and disrupt sleep.

- **High-sodium processed meals** — these strain your kidneys and elevate blood pressure, mimicking stress responses.

Don't see this as loss — see it as making room for clarity. Your body can't reset in a cluttered environment, and neither can your pantry.

What to Stock: The Cortisol-Calming Essentials

Now fill your space with foods that whisper calm into your cells:

- **Leafy greens and cruciferous vegetables:** spinach, kale, broccoli, bok choy — rich in magnesium and detox-supportive compounds.
- **Healthy fats:** avocado, olive oil, nuts, and seeds — fuel for hormonal balance and brain calm.
- **Clean proteins:** salmon, eggs, lentils, and grass-fed poultry — support muscle repair and adrenal strength.

- **Whole carbs:** quinoa, oats, sweet potatoes — provide sustained energy without blood sugar chaos.
- **Adaptogenic herbs:** ashwagandha, holy basil, maca powder, and licorice (optional under guidance).
- **Herbal teas:** chamomile, lemon balm, and rooibos — nature's nervous system restorers.
- **Fresh fruit:** especially berries and citrus, for antioxidants and natural sweetness.

Create a pantry that breathes ease — simple, clean, uncluttered. Every item should make you feel nourished before you even touch it.

Morning, Afternoon, and Evening Rituals That Stabilize Cortisol

Your body runs on rhythm, and cortisol is the conductor of

that rhythm. When your day has structure — gentle, not rigid — your hormones follow suit. Let's build the cadence of calm through small, steady rituals.

Morning: Rise, Don't Rush

- **Wake with light, not alarms.** Exposure to natural sunlight helps set your cortisol peak at the right time — in the morning.
- **Hydrate before caffeine.** A glass of lemon water or herbal infusion tells your adrenals you're refreshed, not dehydrated.
- **Eat within an hour of waking.** A balanced breakfast with protein and healthy fat steadies blood sugar.
- **Breathe before screens.** Even two minutes of deep breathing can prevent that early cortisol surge triggered by digital overwhelm.

Mantra: "I will not chase my day; I will flow with it."

Afternoon: Refuel and Recenter

- **Eat a real lunch.** Skipping it tells your body you're in famine. Choose calming foods — grilled salmon, greens, quinoa.

- **Take a 10-minute movement break.** Gentle stretching, walking, or stepping outside resets the nervous system and improves focus.

- **Hydrate again.** Add a pinch of sea salt to your water if you feel depleted — it supports adrenal minerals.

- **Check your energy, not your to-do list**. Notice when your energy dips and adjust instead of pushing harder.

Mantra: "My productivity thrives when my peace does."

Evening: Transition to Restoration

- **Dim lights after sunset.** Signal your brain that cortisol's shift is complete.
- **Trade screens for rituals.** Try journaling, tea, or quiet reading.
- **Eat early and lightly.** Give your body space to rest, not digest.
- **Reflect, don't replay.** End the day by listing three things you're grateful for — it gently lowers cortisol through emotional release.

Mantra: "Rest is not the end of progress; it is part of it."

Gentle Introduction to Hydration, Herbal Teas, and Deep Breathing

Your adrenal glands thrive in an environment of hydration and oxygen — two things we underestimate daily.

Hydration: The Forgotten Detox

Water isn't just about thirst; it regulates blood volume, temperature, and cellular communication. Dehydration is one of the fastest ways to elevate cortisol, as the body interprets it as a survival threat.

Aim for 8–10 cups of filtered water a day, flavored with slices of cucumber, lemon, or mint to make it refreshing and ritualistic.

Remember: consistency matters more than quantity at once. Sip steadily throughout the day rather than chugging occasionally.

Herbal Teas: Nature's Calm in a Cup

Herbal teas are liquid therapy. Each plant carries a gentle pharmacology that soothes the nervous system:

- **Chamomile:** eases anxiety and promotes sleep.
- **Lemon balm:** calms the mind and supports digestion.
- **Tulsi (holy basil):** an adaptogen that lowers cortisol naturally.
- **Peppermint:** cools inflammation and refreshes focus.
- **Rooibos:** caffeine-free and rich in antioxidants that support adrenal repair.

Create your own "tea ritual" — perhaps a morning energizer and an evening unwinder. Let each sip become a signal: *I am safe.*

Deep Breathing: The Body's Built-in Reset

You can't lower cortisol without oxygen. Shallow breathing tells your body to prepare for danger; slow, rhythmic breathing tells it you've survived it.

Try this:

Inhale for 4 counts. Hold for 2. Exhale for 6.

Repeat for one minute before meals or sleep. Each breath rebalances your parasympathetic system — the circuitry of calm.

The Art of Beginning Again

As you prepare your space, your meals, and your mind, remember: healing doesn't demand perfection. It asks for presence.

You're not just starting a detox — you're teaching your body to trust you again. To believe that it doesn't have to run on fear or caffeine.

By the time you finish this chapter, your kitchen will look calmer, your mornings will feel lighter, and your body will begin to hum the quiet rhythm of safety.

That's the real science of reset — not chemistry, but consistency.

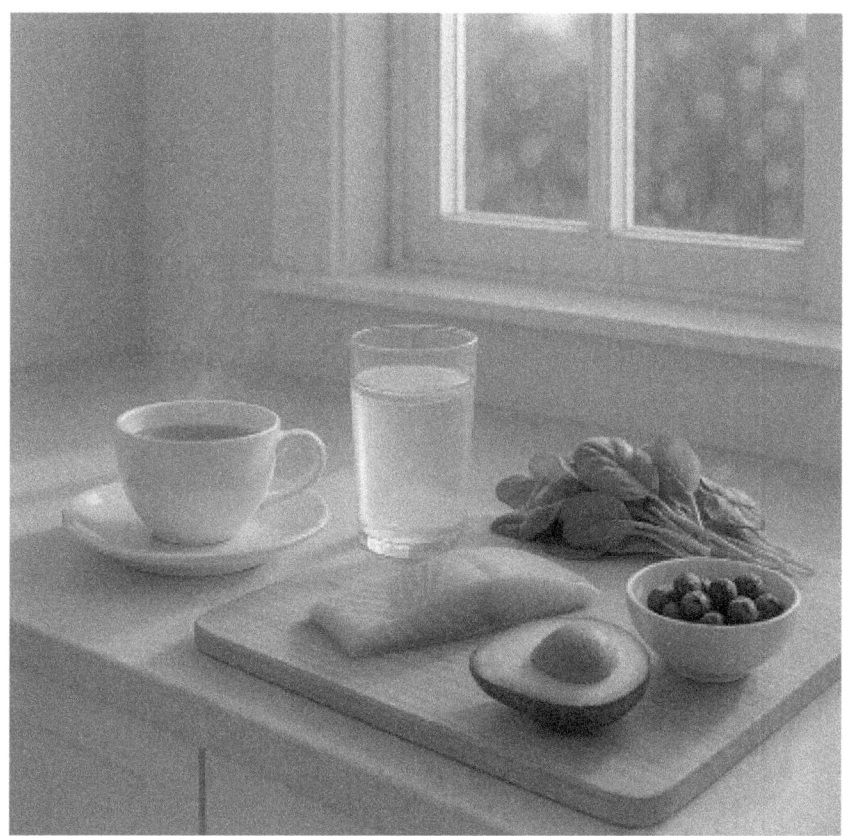

PART II — THE 28-DAY CORTISOL DETOX PLAN

(Each week targets a different stage of hormonal reset.)

Chapter 5

Week 1 — Calm the Chaos: Restoring Inner Balance

When you begin this journey, you may feel like you're unlearning a lifetime of stress. And in many ways, you are.

This first week of your 28-Day Cortisol Detox is not about doing everything perfectly — it's about slowing down enough to notice what your body has been trying to tell you all along. Fatigue, cravings, restless nights — these are not failures; they're signals. Week 1 is about listening, nourishing, and re-teaching your body the language of calm.

Every meal you eat, every breath you take, and every pause you allow becomes part of your reset. This week's focus: **lowering cortisol spikes through balanced meals and rest** — the foundation of everything that follows.

The Purpose of Week One

You can't heal in chaos.

When your body constantly perceives danger — from deadlines, late-night scrolling, skipped meals, or caffeine overload — cortisol remains high, hijacking your energy and mood. The goal this week is to turn that alarm off.

Instead of forcing drastic change, you'll make small, sustainable adjustments that retrain your nervous system to trust you again. The secret isn't intensity — it's consistency.

Think of this week as clearing the storm before rebuilding the house.

Your 7-Day Meal Rhythm

Each day this week follows a calm, predictable rhythm.

You're not counting calories or following strict rules — you're creating hormonal safety through stability. Balanced meals regulate blood sugar, and stable blood sugar keeps cortisol quiet.

Here's what your daily flow will look like:

Morning — Ground Your Energy

- **Fiber-rich breakfast:** Oats with chia seeds, cinnamon, almond butter, and a few berries.

  Why it helps: Fiber slows glucose absorption, preventing early cortisol surges.

- **Optional drink:** Green tea — gentler than coffee, rich in L-theanine to calm the nervous system.
- **Morning ritual:**

  Sit for five minutes before eating. Breathe deeply. Whisper gratitude for your food.

That single moment of presence tells your body: It's safe to digest.

Midday — Sustain and Soothe

- **Protein-balanced lunch:** Grilled salmon, spinach, and quinoa drizzled with olive oil and lemon.

    Why it helps: Omega-3s in salmon reduce inflammation and calm the adrenal glands.

- **Low-sugar snack:** A handful of pumpkin seeds or almonds.

    Why it helps: Magnesium and zinc restore adrenal minerals depleted by stress.

Evening — Ease Into Rest

- **Calming dinner:** Baked chicken or tofu with steamed broccoli and sweet potatoes.

Why it helps: Complex carbs in sweet potatoes gently lower cortisol and support melatonin production.

- **Herbal tea:** Chamomile or lemon balm before bed — your nightly reminder to unwind.

Each meal this week is designed not only to nourish but to retrain. You are teaching your hormones a new rhythm — one that rises with sunlight and rests with the moon.

Key Foods for Week One

Food is the foundation of peace. This week, focus on these calming heroes:

1. Salmon — The Anti-Stress Protein

Rich in omega-3 fatty acids, salmon lowers inflammation, reduces anxiety symptoms, and supports serotonin balance. It also helps regulate the body's response to stress by reducing the intensity of cortisol release.

2. Spinach — The Magnesium Miracle

Spinach replenishes magnesium, one of the first minerals depleted during chronic stress. It supports muscle relaxation, nerve function, and balanced sleep patterns.

3. Pumpkin Seeds — Nature's Adrenal Tonic

Tiny but mighty, pumpkin seeds are packed with magnesium, zinc, and tryptophan — nutrients essential for calming the nervous system and supporting better sleep.

4. Green Tea — Gentle Energy, Calm Focus

Unlike coffee, green tea's L-theanine content promotes mental alertness without triggering cortisol spikes. It delivers focus with serenity — the perfect companion for your mornings or midafternoons.

Include at least two of these foods daily. Over time, you'll notice subtle shifts: steadier energy, softer cravings, and a quieter mind.

Stress Relief Rituals for This Week

Hormone balance doesn't happen through food alone. It happens in the quiet moments you create between the chaos.

1. Journaling for Release

Every evening, take five minutes to write. Don't overthink — just release.

Ask yourself:

- "What drained my energy today?"
- "What restored it?"
- "What am I grateful for right now?"

This isn't about perfection or eloquence — it's about permission. Writing slows the mind and allows emotions to move instead of stagnate. Over time, journaling becomes emotional detox — the mental version of your cortisol reset.

2. Bedtime Screen Breaks

The glow of your phone is more powerful than you think. Blue light tells your brain it's daytime, suppressing melatonin and keeping cortisol elevated long after sunset.

Commit to a **digital sunset** — turning off screens at least 60 minutes before bed.

Replace the scroll with something slower:

- Stretching in dim light
- Sipping herbal tea
- Reading something uplifting or reflective

This simple act can restore sleep quality within days — and deep sleep is one of the most powerful cortisol regulators there is.

3. The Evening Pause

Before bed, stand by a window or step outside. Look at the night sky, even if it's cloudy.

Inhale deeply, exhale slowly, and remind yourself: The day is over. I can rest now.

That conscious exhale tells your body that the danger has passed — even if all that threatened you was another busy day.

A Gentle Reminder

You don't have to earn rest. You deserve it.

This week isn't a race or a cleanse — it's a return. A return to slow mornings, steady meals, unhurried nights, and the steady beat of a heart that remembers calm.

Your body has been waiting for this moment — the permission to pause.

And every balanced meal, every mindful sip, every quiet breath will begin the work of unwinding years of survival mode.

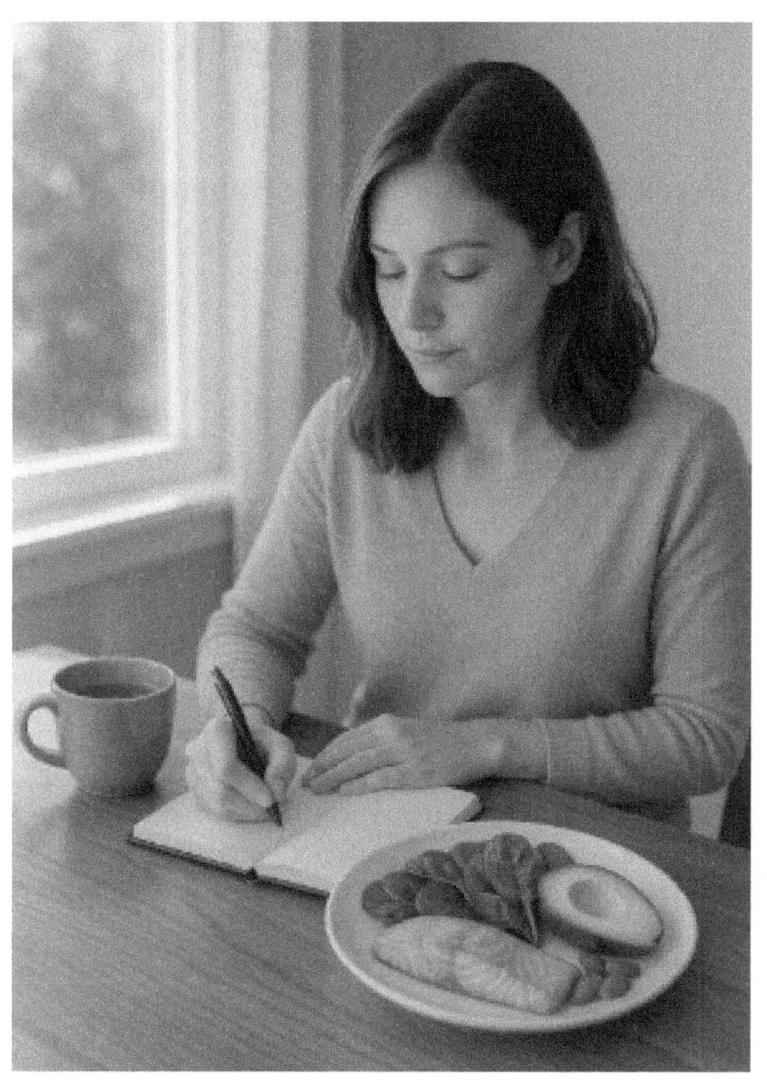

Chapter 6

Week 2 — Nourish to Heal: Rebuilding the Gut and Adrenals

Healing never happens in chaos; it unfolds quietly in rhythm.

If Week 1 was about calming the storm, Week 2 is about repair — mending the deeper structures that stress has worn thin: your gut and your adrenals.

This week is where nutrition meets restoration. The foods and rituals you'll practice here rebuild what chronic stress slowly depleted — digestive strength, hormonal balance, and the subtle sense of safety that allows your body to heal instead of defend.

The body you live in has an extraordinary capacity for renewal. All it needs is nourishment, consistency, and the message that the battle is finally over.

Why Gut and Adrenal Healing Go Hand in Hand

The gut and adrenal glands are partners in resilience.

When your gut is inflamed or imbalanced, it sends distress signals that activate your stress response. Likewise, when cortisol remains high from chronic stress, digestion weakens, leading to bloating, cravings, fatigue, and nutrient loss — a vicious loop.

Healing one system means nurturing the other.

Your **gut** is where nutrients absorb and immune defenses strengthen.

Your **adrenals** control how your body reacts to life's pressures.

When both systems are cared for, energy flows evenly, sleep deepens, and calm begins to feel natural again.

This week, your meals, habits, and breathing will do exactly that: teach your body how to rest and rebuild.

The Focus of Week Two: Nourishment as Medicine

The purpose here isn't to "cleanse" — it's **to feed the systems that heal you.**

Every sip of broth, every mindful breath, every leafy green is a small act of repair.

Your cortisol is now beginning to level from Week 1's reset; it's time to give your body what it needs to rebuild — nutrients, rest, and rhythm.

You'll achieve this through three key practices:

1. Gut-healing, nutrient-dense meals
2. Morning adaptogenic smoothies
3. Self-care habits that slow the stress response at its root

Gut-Friendly Meals: Bone Broth, Fermented Foods, and Leafy Greens

1. Bone Broth – The Liquid Healer

Bone broth is more than a comforting soup — it's a mineral elixir for your gut and adrenals. Rich in collagen, gelatin, and amino acids like glycine and glutamine, it soothes the gut lining, supports digestion, and helps reduce inflammation.

Have a small cup mid-morning or in the evening before dinner. Add a pinch of sea salt or turmeric for flavor and extra adrenal support.

If you're plant-based, replace bone broth with **vegetable broth** made from seaweed, mushrooms, and herbs — it still carries minerals and grounding warmth.

Purpose: To replenish and seal the digestive lining while hydrating your adrenal glands with natural electrolytes.

2. Fermented Foods – Your Gut's New Allies

Stress changes the gut microbiome, reducing the diversity of healthy bacteria that help you absorb nutrients and manage inflammation.

Fermented foods repopulate that microbiome, improving digestion and calming the gut-brain axis — the invisible link between your belly and your mood.

Add small portions of:

- Sauerkraut or kimchi — tangy and rich in probiotics.
- Plain kefir or unsweetened yogurt — supportive to both gut and hormonal balance.
- Kombucha (lightly fermented) — sip occasionally for natural probiotics, not as a sugary beverage.

Purpose: To retrain your gut to process food with ease and restore inner balance between bacteria and stress hormones.

3. Leafy Greens – The Mineral Restorers

By now, you'll recognize how magnesium-rich greens like spinach, kale, and Swiss chard show up repeatedly. That's no coincidence.

Magnesium and folate — abundant in these greens — are the two nutrients cortisol depletes most. Without them, your energy dips, mood wavers, and sleep suffers.

Add a handful of greens to every meal — in smoothies, soups, or light sautés.

They act like natural antidepressants for your cells.

Purpose: To restore micronutrients drained by stress, regulate bowel movement, and enhance cellular oxygenation for adrenal recovery.

Morning Smoothies with Adaptogens

Your mornings now move from survival to vitality.

These smoothies are liquid calm — fast, nourishing, and formulated to deliver energy without caffeine or sugar.

Base Formula:

- 1 cup almond milk or oat milk
- ½ banana or ½ avocado (creamy texture + potassium)
- 1 tablespoon nut butter (healthy fat for satiety)
- 1 handful spinach or kale
- 1 scoop protein powder (pea, hemp, or collagen-based)
- ½ teaspoon adaptogen (Ashwagandha, Maca, or Holy Basil)
- 1 pinch cinnamon or ginger
- Ice or berries as desired

Blend until smooth and sip slowly — not on the go, but as part of your morning calm ritual.

Why Adaptogens Matter:

Adaptogens are plants that help the body adapt to physical and emotional stress. They regulate cortisol rather than suppress it — teaching your body to respond to pressure with steadiness instead of panic.

This small daily ritual balances blood sugar, prevents morning crashes, and helps keep cortisol aligned with your circadian rhythm. It's the perfect bridge from nourishment to serenity.

Mindful Breathing and Self-Care Habits

Nutrition can rebuild the body — but breath rebuilds the nervous system.

Even the most nutrient-rich meals can't reach full potential if your nervous system is still living in overdrive. Mindful breathing and self-care restore this vital connection.

1. The 4–2–6 Breath

Breathe in for 4 counts, hold for 2, and exhale for 6.

This simple ratio extends the exhale, activating your parasympathetic nervous system — the body's "calm switch."

Do it before meals, during stress, or whenever you feel tension rise. Over time, your body will learn that exhalation means safety.

2. The Slow Morning

Replace morning rush with intention. Wake 15 minutes earlier. Sit with your tea. Journal a single sentence about what you're grateful for.

This quiet practice stabilizes cortisol's natural morning rise — turning it from a spike into a steady curve of energy.

3. The Afternoon Pause

After lunch, take a brief walk or simply step outside. Let natural light hit your eyes and fresh air fill your lungs. Movement improves digestion and helps clear stress hormones circulating in your blood.

4. The Self-Care Reset

Each evening, choose one act of kindness for yourself — a warm bath, herbal tea, gentle stretching, or simply silence. The goal isn't luxury; it's permission. You're reminding your body that rest is productive.

A Deeper Truth About Healing

Healing the gut and adrenals is not about adding endless supplements or chasing trends. It's about alignment — syncing your food, breath, and daily choices with what your biology has been craving: peace, rhythm, and nourishment.

Each meal you prepare this week is an act of faith in your body's wisdom.

Each breath you take says, I'm not at war with my own energy anymore.

Each ritual — no matter how small — becomes a brick in the foundation of your recovery.

Week 2 is where healing begins to feel real.

Your energy will begin to stabilize. Your sleep will deepen. And most importantly, you'll start to feel that lightness that comes when your body no longer fears the day.

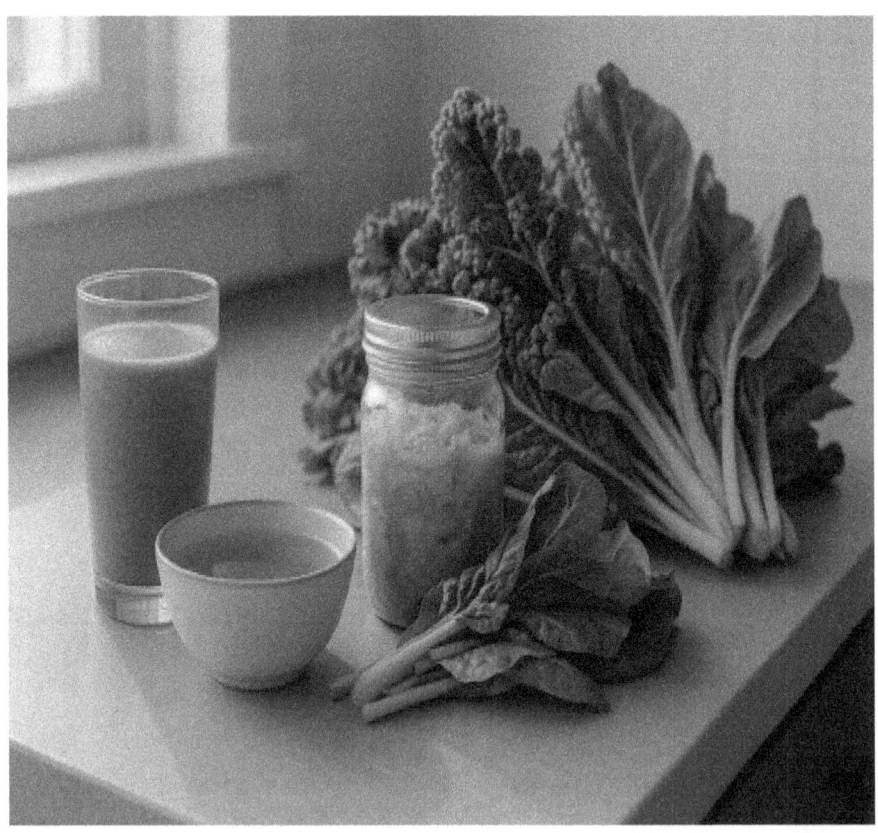

Chapter 7

Week 3 — Revitalize Energy: From Burnout to Brilliance

There is a moment in every healing journey when the fog begins to lift.

The heaviness in the limbs softens. The morning feels a little less like a battle. You notice pockets of lightness in your day — moments when you breathe without effort, when your thoughts feel clearer, when fatigue no longer drags behind you like a shadow.

Week 3 is that moment.

The body is shifting from depletion to replenishment, from burnout to brilliance.

Your cortisol levels have begun to stabilize, inflammation has eased, digestion has strengthened — and now, your energy system can finally receive nourishment instead of just surviving. This week is all about **building vitality**, the kind that feels steady, grounded, and sustainable.

This is not the jittery "energy" caffeine gives.

It's the quiet sensation of having enough — enough fuel, enough breath, enough resilience to move through your day with confidence and clarity.

The Focus of Week 3

Natural ways to restore energy and fight fatigue.

This week reintroduces rhythm to your life — energizing mornings, meaningful movement, a stabilized mood, and a sleep cycle aligned with nature. You're guiding your body back to its innate blueprint: wake with the sun, rise with ease, move with purpose, and rest without resistance.

Your pillars this week:

1. **Energizing breakfasts that stabilize and uplift**

2. Moderate, cortisol-friendly exercises
3. Resetting your sleep cycle with natural cues

Energizing Breakfasts: High-Protein, Slow-Carb Fuel

Fatigue is often not a lack of motivation — it's a lack of stable blood sugar.

Week 3 breakfasts are engineered for metabolic calm and sustained fuel, not quick bursts that collapse into crashes.

The key is **protein + slow carbohydrates + healthy fats**. Together, they give:

- Steady glucose release
- Balanced cortisol rhythm
- Reduced cravings
- Sharper focus
- Longer-lasting energy

Here are your Week 3 hero breakfasts:

1. Savory Protein Bowl

- Grilled salmon or eggs
- Spinach sautéed in olive oil
- Half an avocado
- A small scoop of quinoa

Why it works:

Rich in omega-3s, magnesium, and complete proteins, this bowl stabilizes the morning cortisol peak and nourishes mitochondria — your cells' energy engines.

2. Greek Yogurt Parfait with Slow Carbs

- Unsweetened Greek yogurt
- Handful of berries
- Two tablespoons pumpkin seeds or walnuts

- A drizzle of raw honey (optional)

Why it works:

The combination of protein and fiber slows digestion, supports gut health, and provides antioxidants that combat stress-related fatigue.

3. Warm Cinnamon Oats with Almond Butter

- Steel-cut oats
- Cinnamon
- Almond butter
- Chia seeds

Why it works:

Oats release glucose slowly, preventing mid-morning crashes. Cinnamon stabilizes blood sugar, while chia seeds add omega-3s and satiating fiber.

4. Power Smoothie

- Spinach
- Pea or collagen protein
- Half a banana
- Almond milk
- Teaspoon of maca root (an energizing adaptogen)

Why it works:

Maca supports adrenal function and hormonal equilibrium, lifting energy without overstimulation.

These breakfasts are not just meals; they're morning medicine — the kind that tells your body: *You are safe. You have enough. Begin with strength.*

Movement for Vitality: Yoga, Walking & Stretching

Burnout does not mean your body is broken — it means it has been trying too hard for too long.

The solution isn't intense exercise; it's movement that communicates safety while stimulating blood flow, oxygen, and endorphins.

This week's movement plan is intentionally moderate, designed to energize without elevating cortisol.

1. Yoga: Move with Breath

10–20 minutes each morning or evening

Focus on poses that open the chest, hips, and spine

Benefits:

- Lengthens tight muscles contracted by stress
- Increases circulation and oxygenation
- Reduces cortisol and shifts the body into parasympathetic calm
- Quiets anxious thoughts

Even a few sun salutations can ignite a spark of vitality

from within.

2. Walking: The Most Underrated Energy Medicine

Aim for 20–30 minutes daily

Preferably outdoors

Benefits:

- Increases serotonin and dopamine
- Enhances mitochondrial energy production
- Improves digestion
- Clears mental fog
- Synchronizes circadian rhythms

With each step, your body remembers its natural rhythm.

3. Stretching: Flexibility for the

Nervous System

5 minutes before bed or upon waking

Focus on neck, shoulders, hips, and back

Benefits:

- Releases stored tension
- Improves circulation
- Signals safety
- Helps reduce nighttime cortisol

Fatigue often hides in stiffness. When your body softens, energy flows more freely.

Resetting the Sleep Cycle with Natural Cues

Energy is not created during the day — it is borrowed from the night before.

To revitalize energy, you must repair your relationship

with sleep. That means aligning your internal clock with the signals nature has used for thousands of years: light, darkness, temperature, stillness.

Here's how Week 3 gently resets sleep:

1. Morning Sunlight Exposure

Within 10–20 minutes of waking

Sit near a window or step outside

Why it works:

- Sets your cortisol peak at the right time (morning, not evening)
- Boosts serotonin, which later converts to melatonin
- Improves energy and mood throughout the day

Sunlight is nature's original stimulant — gentle, steady, and rhythmic.

2. Evening Wind-Down Ritual

Avoid screens 60 minutes before bed

Dim lights

Sip chamomile or lemon balm tea

Light stretching or slow breathing

Why it works:

- Artificial light tells your brain it's still daytime.
- Darkness whispers, "It's time to rest."

3. Cool, Quiet, Comfort-Promoting Bedroom

Lower room temperature

Keep noise minimal

Use soft, warm lighting

Why it works:

- Cortisol decreases in cooler environments, allowing melatonin to rise naturally.

4. The 10-3-2-1-0 Rule (Modified for Stress Recovery)

10 hours before bed: No caffeine

3 hours before bed: No heavy meals

2 hours before bed: Light activity only

1 hour before bed: No screens

0: Number of times you hit snooze

This creates a predictable pattern that your nervous system can rely on — and safety creates sleep.

The Beauty of Week 3

This week teaches you a profound truth:

Energy doesn't need to be forced. It can be invited.

As your cortisol rhythm steadies, inflammation decreases, and your gut absorbs nutrients more efficiently, your body slowly emerges from survival mode.

You'll feel:

- A clearer mind
- A lighter body
- Improved stamina
- More stable moods
- A sense of returning to yourself

You are not just gaining energy — you are reclaiming the brilliance that stress once dimmed.

Week 3 is your turning point. Your body is no longer merely coping — it is rebuilding.

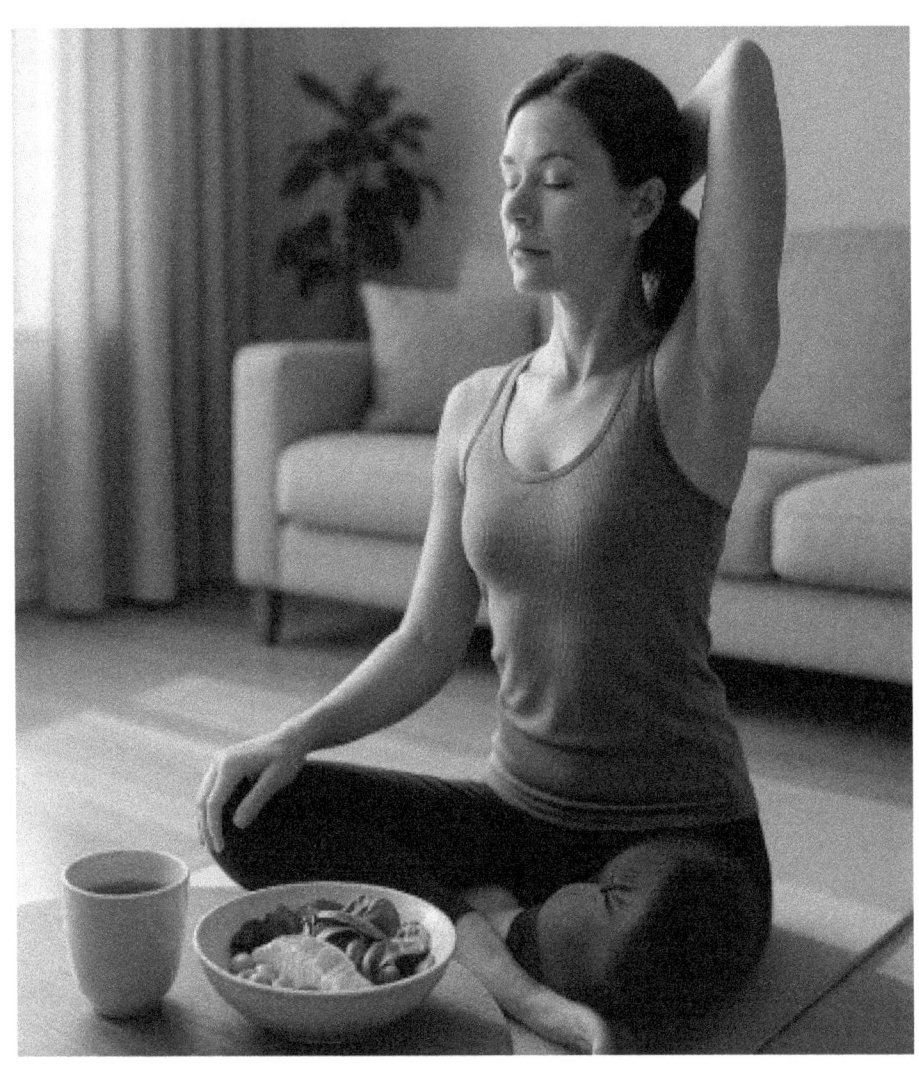

Chapter 8

Week 4 — Sustain and Strengthen: Living Stress-Free Beyond Detox

By now, something important has shifted.

Stress no longer feels like a constant background noise. Your body responds faster to rest. Your mind feels steadier. Energy flows more naturally, without force.

Week 4 is not an ending — it's a transition.

This is where the detox becomes a lifestyle, where calm stops being something you do and starts becoming something you are.

The focus this week is **maintenance with freedom**. You are learning how to live fully — enjoying food, managing pressure, navigating emotions — without triggering cortisol overload again. The goal is not perfection, but resilience.

This is how balance becomes permanent.

The Focus of Week 4

Maintaining hormonal balance and long-term calm.

This week teaches you how to:

- Reintroduce flexibility without fear
- Handle real-life stressors without spiraling
- Turn everyday routines into wellness rituals

You are no longer detoxing from stress — you are living beyond it.

Reintroducing Occasional Treats Without Triggering Cortisol

Restriction creates stress.

And stress — even from "clean eating" — raises cortisol

just as surely as sugar or caffeine does.

The key to long-term balance is intentional flexibility.

How to Reintroduce Treats Safely

Treats don't disrupt cortisol — patterns do. One mindful indulgence won't harm your hormones. Chronic guilt, binge-restrict cycles, and blood sugar crashes will.

Follow these principles:

1. Never eat treats on an empty stomach

Always pair treats with protein or healthy fats. This stabilizes blood sugar and prevents cortisol spikes.

2. Choose quality over quantity

A small piece of dark chocolate, a homemade dessert, or a favorite meal enjoyed slowly is far less stressful to the body than mindless snacking.

3. Eat without guilt

Shame activates the stress response. Enjoyment deactivates it. Eat treats consciously and move on.

4. Return to rhythm the next meal

Balance is built over days, not moments.

When food is no longer emotionally charged, cortisol stays calm.

Managing Deadlines, Relationships, and Emotions Mindfully

Life doesn't slow down just because your hormones are healing.

Deadlines still arrive. Relationships still test you. Emotions still rise.

The difference now is **how you respond**.

1. Deadlines Without Overdrive

Stress spikes when urgency replaces intention.

Before reacting:

- Pause for one breath
- Ask: *"What's the next calm step?"*
- Break tasks into single actions

This keeps cortisol from escalating unnecessarily.

2. Relationships Without Emotional Exhaustion

Not every emotion needs immediate resolution.

Practice:

- Listening without fixing
- Pausing before responding
- Allowing silence

Emotional boundaries protect your nervous system just as much as sleep and nutrition.

3. Emotions as Signals, Not Threats

Anxiety, frustration, or sadness are messages — not emergencies.

Instead of suppressing emotions:

- Name them
- Breathe through them
- Let them pass

This prevents emotional buildup that quietly fuels cortisol over time.

Turning Daily Routines Into Wellness Rituals

The most powerful stress-management tools are the ones you already do every day.

Morning Rituals

- Wake with light
- Hydrate before caffeine
- Eat a balanced breakfast
- Set one intention for the day

This aligns cortisol with its natural morning rise.

Midday Anchors

- Eat without rushing
- Step outside briefly
- Stretch or breathe

These pauses prevent cumulative stress.

Evening Wind-Down

- Dim lights
- Limit screens
- Reflect on what went well
- Sleep consistently

This trains cortisol to fall naturally at night.

Rituals turn routine into regulation.

Your New Relationship With Stress

Stress will still exist — but it no longer owns you.

You now understand:

- How to calm your body through food
- How to stabilize energy naturally
- How to rest without guilt
- How to respond instead of react

This is what sustainable wellness looks like.

Not extreme.

Not rigid.

Not exhausting.

Just balanced, aware, and deeply human.

Beyond the 28 Days

You don't need to "stay on" this plan forever.

You are the plan now.

Use this reset whenever life feels heavy again — after travel, burnout, emotional upheaval, or change. Return to the rhythms you've learned. Trust your body's cues.

Adjust with compassion.

Your hormones don't need control.

They need cooperation.

And you've learned how to give them exactly that.

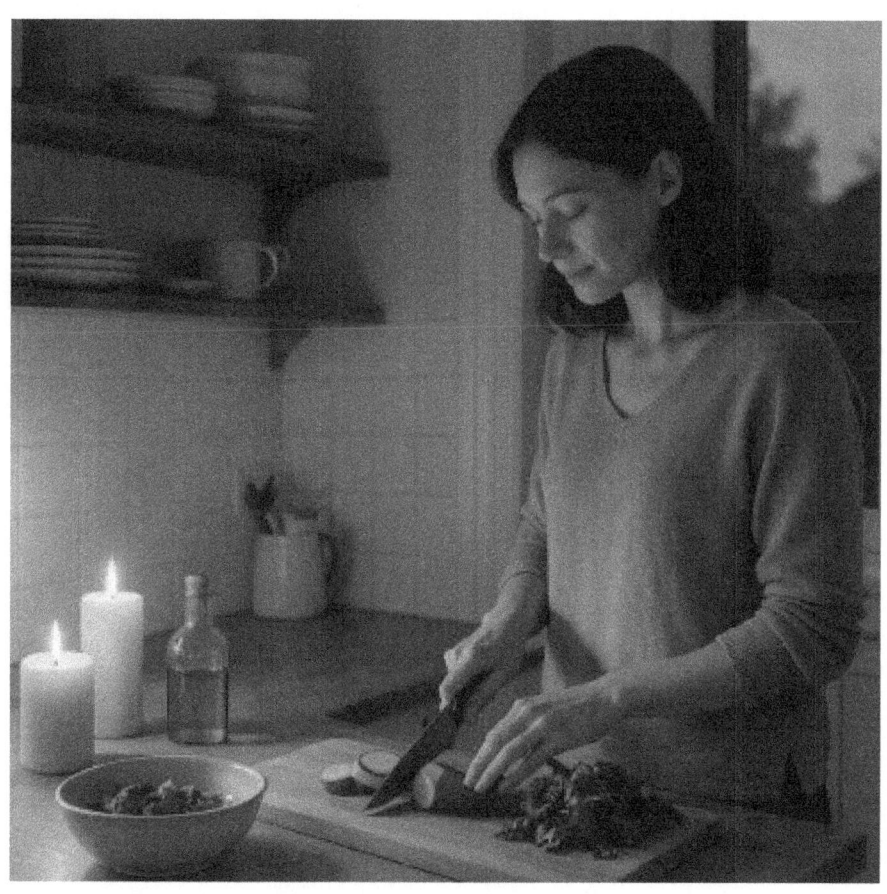

PART III — RECIPES & RITUALS FOR HORMONAL BALANCE

Chapter 9

Cortisol-Lowering Recipes for Every Meal

By now, you understand something powerful: food is not just nourishment — it is instruction.

Every meal you eat teaches your body either urgency or ease. Scarcity or safety. Stress or stability.

This chapter is where theory becomes tangible. Where cortisol balance moves from concept to plate.

The recipes in this section are designed with one purpose: **to steady blood sugar, calm the nervous system, and support your body's natural rhythm from morning to night**. Nothing extreme. Nothing complicated. Just deeply supportive food that works with your hormones, not against them.

Think of this chapter as your everyday toolkit — meals

you can return to again and again whenever stress creeps back in.

Breakfasts to Steady Blood Sugar

Morning meals set the hormonal tone for the entire day.

When breakfast is skipped, sugary, or caffeine-heavy, cortisol rises fast and stays elevated. The goal here is grounded energy, not stimulation.

Spinach & Egg Breakfast Skillet

Sauté fresh spinach in olive oil, add eggs, and finish with pumpkin seeds and sea salt.

Why it works:

Protein stabilizes blood sugar, spinach replenishes magnesium, and healthy fats prevent cortisol spikes.

Warm Cinnamon Oats with Almond Butter

Steel-cut oats cooked slowly, stirred with cinnamon and

topped with almond butter and berries.

Why it works:

Slow-digesting carbs provide sustained energy, while cinnamon improves glucose control.

Greek Yogurt Calm Bowl

Unsweetened Greek yogurt topped with walnuts, chia seeds, and a drizzle of raw honey.

Why it works:

Protein plus omega-3s support adrenal recovery and reduce inflammation.

Green Morning Smoothie

Spinach, avocado, pea or collagen protein, almond milk, and a pinch of ginger.

Why it works:

This combination nourishes without overwhelming digestion and supports cortisol's natural morning rise.

Nourishing Lunches That Fuel Calm

Lunch should restore you — not weigh you down or leave you wired and tired. These meals keep energy steady through the afternoon, when cortisol imbalances often surface.

Salmon & Quinoa Nourish Bowl

Grilled salmon, quinoa, leafy greens, olive oil, and lemon.

Why it works:

Omega-3s reduce inflammation and cortisol reactivity; quinoa provides slow, stable energy.

Lentil & Vegetable Stew

Lentils simmered with carrots, celery, garlic, and herbs.

Why it works:

Fiber supports gut health, which directly influences stress hormones.

Avocado & Chicken Power Salad

Mixed greens topped with roasted chicken, avocado, pumpkin seeds, and olive oil dressing.

Why it works:

Balanced macros prevent the afternoon energy crash that often triggers stress eating.

Bone Broth Vegetable Bowl

Warm bone broth poured over steamed vegetables and rice or sweet potato.

Why it works:

Minerals and collagen support adrenal recovery and digestion.

Soothing Dinners for Better Sleep

Evening meals should signal safety, not stimulation. Heavy, late, or sugary dinners can keep cortisol elevated at night and disrupt sleep.

Baked Salmon with Sweet Potatoes

Salmon roasted with herbs, served alongside baked sweet potatoes and greens.

Why it works:

Complex carbs gently lower evening cortisol and support melatonin production.

Vegetable Stir-Fry with Tofu

Lightly cooked vegetables with tofu and ginger, served over brown rice.

Why it works:

Easy digestion and plant-based protein reduce nighttime stress on the body.

Chicken & Root Vegetable Tray Bake

Chicken roasted with carrots, parsnips, and olive oil.

Why it works:

Grounding foods calm the nervous system and promote deep rest.

Simple Soup & Greens

A warm bowl of soup with sautéed spinach or kale.

Why it works:

Warm foods activate the parasympathetic nervous system, preparing the body for sleep.

Herbal Teas, Snacks, and Smoothies

These are the gentle bridges between meals — designed to prevent cortisol spikes without constant grazing.

Herbal Teas for Calm

- **Chamomile:** Promotes relaxation and sleep

- **Lemon balm:** Reduces anxiety and digestive tension
- **Tulsi (Holy Basil):** Adaptogen that lowers cortisol naturally
- **Rooibos:** Caffeine-free antioxidant support

Sip slowly. Tea is as much ritual as nourishment.

Low-Stress Snacks

- Pumpkin seeds
- Almonds or walnuts
- Apple slices with nut butter
- Greek yogurt
- A small square of dark chocolate

Rule of calm snacking: Always pair carbs with protein or fat.

Adaptogenic Smoothies

Almond milk, protein powder, berries, spinach, and a small amount of ashwagandha or maca.

Why it works:

Adaptogens help regulate — not suppress — the stress response.

Your Cortisol-Calming Weekly Recipe Rotation

This weekly rotation is built around one simple principle:

rhythm creates safety, and safety lowers cortisol.

Instead of constantly deciding what to eat (which quietly raises stress), this rotation removes decision fatigue while keeping meals varied, nourishing, and enjoyable. You can repeat this same weekly rhythm throughout the detox — or return to it anytime life feels overwhelming.

Each day follows a predictable pattern:

- **Breakfast:** Grounded energy
- **Lunch:** Steady focus
- **Dinner:** Nervous-system calm
- **Snack/Tea:** Gentle support between meals

Monday – Reset & Ground

Breakfast:

Spinach & egg breakfast skillet with pumpkin seeds

Lunch:

Salmon and quinoa nourish bowl with olive oil and lemon

Dinner:

Baked chicken with sweet potatoes and steamed broccoli

Snack / Tea:

Handful of almonds + chamomile tea

Why this day works:

Starts the week by replenishing magnesium and protein, calming the adrenal response after the weekend.

Tuesday – Digest & Restore

Breakfast:

Warm cinnamon oats with almond butter and berries

Lunch:

Lentil and vegetable stew

Dinner:

Vegetable stir-fry with tofu and brown rice

Snack / Tea:

Greek yogurt with walnuts + lemon balm tea

Why this day works:

Fiber-rich meals support gut healing, which directly

reduces cortisol signaling.

Wednesday – Energize Gently

Breakfast:

Green morning smoothie with protein and avocado

Lunch:

Avocado and grilled chicken power salad

Dinner:

Salmon with roasted root vegetables

Snack / Tea:

Apple slices with nut butter + green tea (earlier in the day)

Why this day works:

Boosts energy midweek without caffeine overload or sugar crashes.

Thursday – Balance & Focus

Breakfast:

Greek yogurt calm bowl with chia seeds and honey

Lunch:

Bone broth vegetable bowl with rice or sweet potato

Dinner:

Simple soup with sautéed kale

Snack / Tea:

Pumpkin seeds + rooibos tea

Why this day works:

Supports adrenal recovery while keeping digestion light and efficient.

Friday – Support & Soothe

Breakfast:

Savory protein bowl with eggs, spinach, and quinoa

Lunch:

Salmon salad with olive oil dressing

Dinner:

Chicken and root vegetable tray bake

Snack / Tea:

Dark chocolate square + chamomile tea

Why this day works:

Allows a gentle sense of indulgence without triggering cortisol spikes.

Saturday – Nourish & Enjoy

Breakfast:

Warm oats or smoothie of choice

Lunch:

Leftover nourish bowl or lentil stew

Dinner:

Favorite home-cooked meal using whole ingredients

Snack / Tea:

Yogurt or nuts + herbal tea

Why this day works:

Encourages flexibility and enjoyment — critical for long-term hormone balance.

Sunday – Reset & Prepare

Breakfast:

Eggs with leafy greens and avocado

Lunch:

Soup or broth-based meal

Dinner:

Light dinner (vegetables + protein) eaten early

Snack / Tea:

Herbal tea and fruit

Why this day works:

Prepares the body and nervous system for the upcoming week with calm and intention.

How to Use This Rotation for the Entire Detox

- Repeat this same weekly structure for Weeks 1–4, swapping proteins or vegetables as desired
- Keep the meal rhythm, not perfection
- When life gets busy, return to the basics: protein + fiber + healthy fat
- Use leftovers intentionally to reduce stress

This rotation isn't about strict adherence — it's about **predictability**, which is one of the most powerful cortisol-lowering tools you have.

If You Slip or Feel Overwhelmed

Return to:

- Warm breakfast
- Balanced lunch
- Light dinner
- Herbal tea

Your body remembers calm faster than you think.

How to Use This Chapter Long-Term

You don't need to eat perfectly to stay balanced.

You need rhythm.

Return to these meals whenever:

- You feel wired but tired
- Sleep becomes restless
- Cravings increase
- Stress levels rise

These recipes are not a diet — they're a reset button.

Your body remembers calm faster than you think.

A Final Note on Food and Freedom

The most cortisol-lowering ingredient of all is peace.

Eat slowly. Enjoy your meals. Release guilt. Trust your body.

Food works best when it's received in safety.

And now, you know how to create that — every morning, every afternoon, every night.

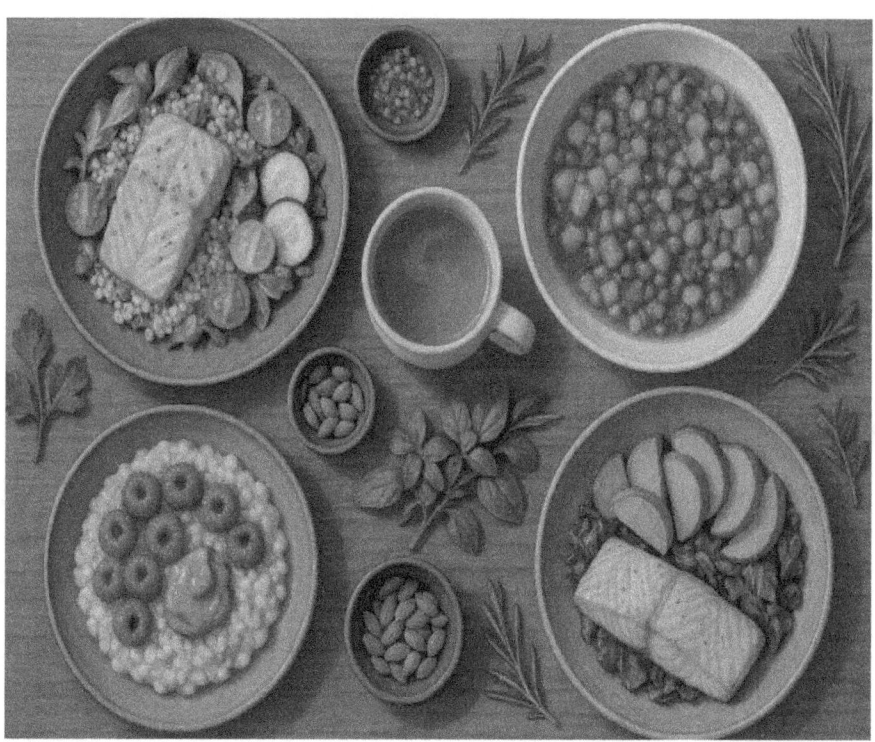

Chapter 10

Stress Detox Rituals and Lifestyle Blueprint

By now, you've learned something most people never do: stress is not just something that happens to you—it's something your body learns how to respond to.

This chapter is where knowledge becomes embodiment.

The meals you've eaten, the sleep you've restored, the energy you've reclaimed—none of it is random. You've been retraining your nervous system. And now, you're ready to build a life that supports calm automatically, without constant effort or willpower.

This chapter gives you a **blueprint**—not a schedule you must obey, but a rhythm you can return to whenever life speeds up.

Breathing Patterns That Reduce

Cortisol in 60 Seconds

Breath is the fastest way to change your stress chemistry. No supplements. No equipment. No time investment.

When cortisol rises, your breathing becomes shallow and fast. When you slow your breath, your body receives an immediate message: the threat has passed.

The 60-Second Cortisol Reset Breath

- Inhale through your nose for 4 seconds
- Hold gently for 2 seconds
- Exhale slowly through your mouth for 6 seconds
- Repeat 5 times

This pattern lengthens the exhale, activating the vagus nerve and shifting your body into parasympathetic mode—the state where healing, digestion, and hormonal balance occur.

Use this:

- Before meals
- During emotional tension
- Before difficult conversations
- Before sleep

One minute can change the entire trajectory of your day.

Journaling, Gratitude, and Emotional Regulation

Stress doesn't only come from deadlines—it comes from **unprocessed emotion**.

When emotions are ignored or suppressed, cortisol stays elevated. When emotions are acknowledged and expressed safely, the nervous system releases them.

Journaling for Regulation (Not Rumination)

This is not about writing pages. It's about clarity.

Each evening, write just **three short lines**:

1. One thing that challenged you today
2. One thing that supported you
3. One thing you're grateful for

This simple practice trains your brain to *complete stress cycles* instead of carrying them into sleep.

Gratitude as a Biological Tool

Gratitude is not spiritual bypassing—it's nervous system training.

When you consciously recognize safety, your brain reduces threat signaling. Over time, this lowers baseline cortisol levels.

Even on difficult days, gratitude doesn't deny reality—it widens it.

Emotional Regulation: Responding

Instead of Reacting

Emotion becomes stressful only when it feels unsafe.

When something triggers you:

- Pause
- Name the emotion
- Breathe
- Respond intentionally

This interrupts the stress loop and prevents cortisol escalation.

You're not trying to eliminate emotion—you're learning how to hold it.

Creating Your Daily "Calm Schedule"

A calm life isn't unstructured—it's **predictable enough to feel safe, flexible enough to feel human**.

Your calm schedule is built around **anchors**, not rules.

Morning Anchor

- Light exposure
- Hydration
- Nourishing breakfast
- One intention

This aligns cortisol with its natural morning rise.

Midday Anchor

- Balanced lunch
- Short walk or breath break
- Reduced multitasking

This prevents the afternoon stress spike most people mistake for "low energy."

Evening Anchor

- Early, light dinner
- Dim lighting
- Screen reduction
- Reflection or stillness

This trains cortisol to fall naturally, allowing deep sleep.

Your schedule doesn't have to be perfect. It just has to be consistent enough for your body to trust it.

Nature Therapy, Grounding, and Mindfulness

Modern stress comes from disconnection—from the body, from rhythm, from the natural world.

Nature restores what stress disrupts.

Nature Therapy

Spending time outdoors lowers cortisol, blood pressure,

and anxiety—even without exercise.

- Walk in sunlight
- Sit under trees
- Open windows
- Touch plants

Your nervous system recognizes nature as safety.

Grounding

Direct contact with the earth—bare feet on grass, sand, or soil—reduces stress signals and inflammation.

Even a few minutes can stabilize energy and mood.

Mindfulness That Fits Real Life

Mindfulness doesn't require meditation cushions or silence.

It looks like:

- Eating without scrolling
- Feeling your feet on the floor

- Pausing before responding
- Breathing before reacting

Mindfulness is presence, not performance.

Your Long-Term Lifestyle Blueprint

You don't need to live stress-free to be hormonally balanced.

You need to live **stress-aware.**

This blueprint works because it's adaptable:

- Use it during busy seasons
- Return to it after burnout
- Lean on it during emotional upheaval

You now know how to:

- Calm your body in minutes
- Eat in a way that supports hormones
- Sleep without forcing rest

- Navigate emotions without overwhelm

That's not a detox—that's mastery.

A Final Reflection

Your body was never broken.

It was responding exactly as it was designed to.

Now, you've given it new instructions—ones rooted in safety, nourishment, rhythm, and compassion.

Stress may visit again.

But it no longer gets to move in.

You have the tools.

You have the awareness.

And most importantly—you have yourself back.

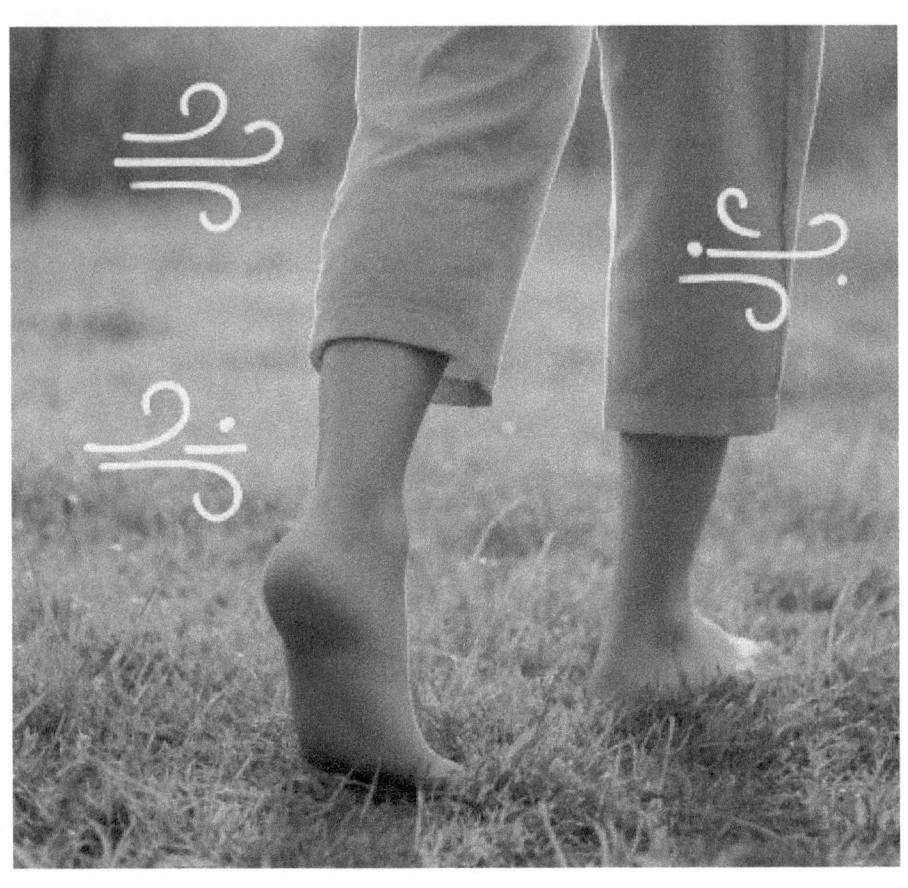

PART IV — LONG-TERM SUCCESS AND SELF-MASTERY

Chapter 11

Rebalancing for Life — Your Post-Detox Maintenance Plan

Finishing a detox can feel strangely vulnerable.

Part of you is proud of what you've rebuilt. Another part quietly wonders, What happens now?

This chapter exists to answer that question gently and honestly.

You are not meant to live in a permanent reset. You are meant to live in a body that knows how to recover quickly, respond wisely, and return to calm without panic or punishment. This is what long-term balance looks like — not control, but awareness.

This chapter gives you the tools **to maintain hormonal balance in real life**, where travel happens, deadlines pile up, emotions rise, and perfection is neither possible nor necessary.

The 80/20 Rule: Flexibility Without Fear

The fastest way to raise cortisol again is rigidity.

The second fastest is guilt.

The **80/20 rule** protects you from both.

Eighty percent of the time, you eat, move, and rest in ways that support calm.

Twenty percent of the time, you live — socially, joyfully, imperfectly.

That flexibility is not a weakness. It's the reason balance lasts.

How to Use the 80/20 Rule in

Practice

Enjoy occasional treats without apology

Attend dinners, celebrations, and travel meals without stress

Choose consistency over intensity

Return to supportive habits at the next meal or the next morning

Your hormones respond to patterns, not moments. One indulgence does not undo balance. Chronic stress about food does.

Freedom is part of hormonal health.

Recognizing Early Signs of Cortisol Flare-Ups

The goal now is not to eliminate stress — it's to catch

imbalance early, before it becomes exhaustion again.

Your body always whispers before it shouts.

Common Early Signals

- Waking tired despite enough sleep
- Increased cravings for sugar or caffeine
- Feeling "wired but tired"
- Shallow breathing or tight shoulders
- Difficulty falling asleep
- Emotional reactivity that feels disproportionate

These are not failures. They are feedback.

When you notice them, don't tighten your rules — **soften your support.**

Your Cortisol Recovery Toolkit

Think of this as your emotional and physical first-aid kit — tools you can reach for on demanding days without overthinking.

Food Reset (24–48 Hours)

- Warm, protein-rich breakfasts
- Balanced lunches
- Light dinners
- Herbal teas
- Adequate hydration

No extremes. Just nourishment.

Nervous System Reset

- 60-second breathing resets
- Short walks outdoors
- Stretching tight areas
- Quiet evenings

Calm the body first. The mind follows.

Emotional Reset

- Journal one page

- Name what you're feeling
- Lower expectations temporarily
- Ask for support if needed

Stress reduces when it's acknowledged.

You don't need all tools every time. One or two is enough to interrupt a flare-up.

Adapting the Plan During Travel, Work Stress, or Life Changes

Life will test your balance. That's not a sign you're doing something wrong — it's where the plan proves it works.

During Travel

- Prioritize protein and hydration
- Walk when possible
- Sleep consistently, even if briefly
- Release food perfection

Movement and rest matter more than ideal meals.

During Work Stress

- Eat regularly, even if meals are simple
- Breathe before meetings
- Take micro-breaks
- Protect sleep

Stress compounds when basic needs are ignored.

During Emotional Seasons

- Lower expectations
- Increase gentleness
- Return to rituals
- Allow rest without guilt

Your body needs compassion most when life is heavy.

The Truth About Long-Term Balance

Balance is not a destination you arrive at and stay forever.

It's a **skill you practice**.

Some weeks will feel effortless.

Others will feel messy.

What matters is that now you know how to return — without fear, without punishment, without starting over.

You don't "fall off" this plan.

You step back into it.

Your New Relationship With Your Body

You no longer need to override your body with willpower.

You listen. You respond. You adjust.

That's the difference between surviving stress and mastering it.

Your body knows how to heal.

You've simply learned how to cooperate.

And that — more than any diet or detox — is what keeps cortisol balanced for life.

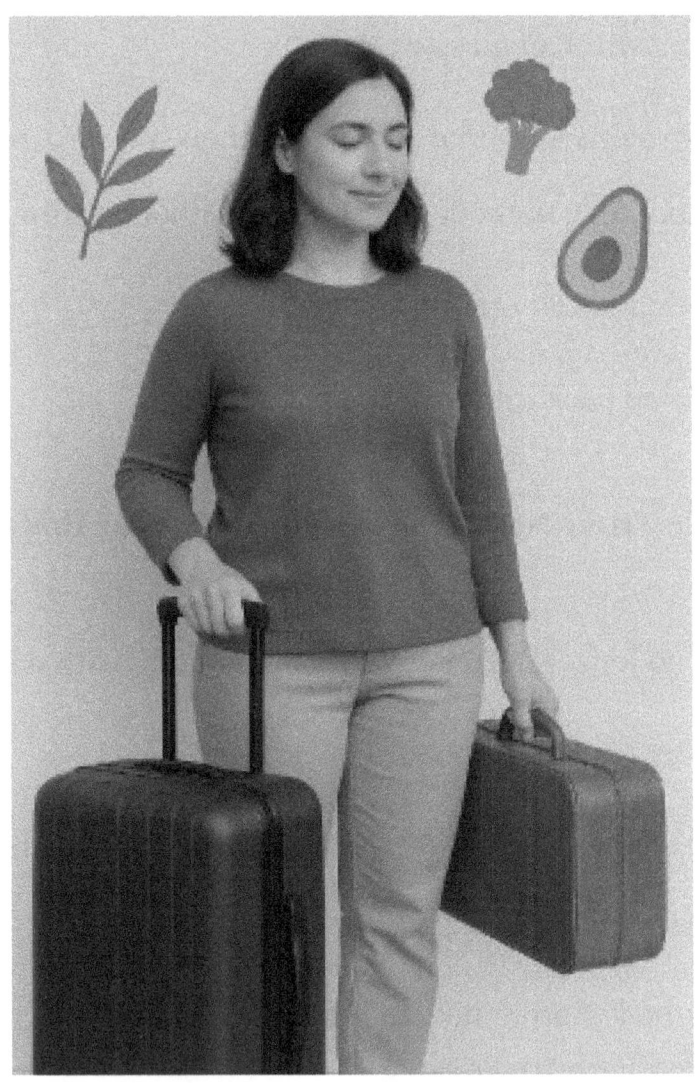

Chapter 12

The 7-Day Emergency Stress Reset

Stress doesn't always announce itself politely.

Sometimes it arrives all at once — through deadlines, emotional upheaval, travel, illness, lack of sleep, or simply too many demands stacked too close together.

This reset exists for those moments.

The **7-Day Emergency Stress Reset** is not about fixing everything. It's about interrupting the stress spiral before it becomes burnout. Think of it as pressing pause on survival mode and guiding your body back to baseline — gently, efficiently, and compassionately.

You can use this reset anytime:

- After an emotionally intense week
- During high-pressure work periods

- After travel or disrupted sleep
- When cravings, fatigue, or anxiety suddenly spike
- When you feel "off" and don't know why

You don't need motivation.

You just need rhythm.

How This Reset Works

For seven days, you will:

- Simplify meals
- Reduce decision fatigue
- Stabilize blood sugar
- Calm the nervous system
- Restore sleep signals

No restriction. No extremes.

Only the essentials your body needs to feel safe again.

The Core Rules (Keep These Simple)

- Eat **three balanced meals** daily
- Include **protein at every meal**
- Drink water consistently
- Move gently
- Protect sleep
- Breathe intentionally

That's it.

Everything else is optional.

Day 1: Stop the Bleeding

Focus: Interrupt cortisol spikes

This day is about containment, not productivity.

Meals

- Warm, protein-rich breakfast

- Simple lunch (soup, bowl, or leftovers)
- Light dinner eaten early

Rituals

- Cancel nonessential commitments
- Reduce caffeine
- Breathe deeply before each meal
- Go to bed early

Reminder:

Today is about safety, not progress.

Day 2: Ground the Body

Focus: Stabilize blood sugar and hydration

Meals

- Oats, eggs, or yogurt for breakfast
- Balanced lunch with protein + fiber
- Root vegetables or rice at dinner

Rituals

- Gentle walk outdoors
- Herbal tea in the evening
- Screens off 60 minutes before bed

Reminder:

Grounded bodies don't panic.

Day 3: Calm the Nervous System

Focus: Parasympathetic activation

Meals

- Repeat simple, familiar foods
- Avoid sugar spikes
- Add magnesium-rich greens

Rituals

- 5 minutes of slow breathing
- Light stretching

- Journaling one page

Prompt:

"What does my body need today?"

Day 4: Restore Energy Gently

Focus: Nourish without stimulation

Meals

- Protein-forward breakfast
- Steady lunch
- Early, calming dinner

Rituals

- Morning sunlight exposure
- Avoid late caffeine
- Short walk or yoga

Reminder:

Energy returns when the body feels safe.

Day 5: Release Emotional Load

Focus: Emotional regulation

Meals

- Comforting, warm foods
- Broth, soup, or stews

Rituals

- Write what you've been carrying
- Name one emotion without fixing it
- Practice self-compassion

Reminder:

Unprocessed emotion keeps cortisol elevated.

Day 6: Rebuild Rhythm

Focus: Predictability

Meals

- Eat at consistent times
- Keep meals simple and familiar

Rituals

- Morning routine
- Midday pause
- Evening wind-down

Reminder:

Rhythm creates trust.

Day 7: Reset Forward

Focus: Integration

Meals

- Balanced, nourishing meals
- No restrictions, no guilt

Rituals

- Reflect on what helped
- Choose 2 habits to carry forward
- Release urgency

Prompt:

"What supports calm in my real life?"

Emergency Reset Shortcuts (When You're Very Overwhelmed)

If seven days feels like too much, do just three things:

1. Eat regularly
2. Breathe slowly
3. Sleep consistently

That alone can prevent a cortisol crash.

What This Reset Is (and Isn't)

This reset is:

- Supportive
- Flexible
- Repeatable
- Compassionate

This reset is not:

- Punitive
- Restrictive
- Perfect
- Another thing to "fail"

You are allowed to need recovery more than once.

A Final Word

Stress does not mean you're weak.

It means you're human.

The difference now is that you know how to return — quickly, kindly, and without starting over.

Use this reset whenever life tightens its grip.

Your body will remember what to do.

And calm will follow.

Chapter 13

Mind Over Cortisol — The Psychology of Lasting Calm

Long before cortisol shows up in bloodwork or belly fat, it begins in thought.

Not every stressful moment is dangerous—but the interpretation of that moment can convince your body that it is. This is where lasting calm is truly built: not by eliminating challenges, but by changing how your mind meets them.

This chapter is about reclaiming authority over your internal world.

The Thought–Stress Connection

Your brain is constantly scanning for threat.

Deadlines. Conversations. Memories. Expectations.

When the brain perceives danger—real or imagined—it activates the stress response. Cortisol rises. Muscles tense. Digestion slows. Sleep becomes shallow.

The body doesn't distinguish between:

- A real emergency
- A fearful thought
- A replayed memory

To your nervous system, thoughts are experiences.

That's why chronic worry, self-criticism, and mental overload can keep cortisol elevated even when life appears calm on the outside.

Awareness is the first interruption.

Rewiring Your Brain's Reaction to

Triggers

Triggers are not flaws. They are learned responses.

Your brain learned them to protect you—but it can also learn to release them.

The Pause Practice

When you feel stress rising:

- Pause
- Name the thought
- Ask: *Is this happening now, or am I imagining a future or replaying the past?*
- Breathe slowly

This simple pause creates space between stimulus and response—the space where cortisol begins to fall.

Over time, your brain rewires itself through repetition. Calm becomes familiar. Safety becomes the default.

Building Emotional Resilience and Inner Peace

Resilience is not toughness.

It is flexibility.

Emotionally resilient people:

Feel deeply

Recover quickly

Don't shame themselves for stress

Don't resist rest

You build resilience by allowing emotion to pass through you instead of trapping it inside.

Crying, journaling, breathing, resting—these are not indulgences. They are biological processes that complete the stress cycle.

Peace isn't numbness.

It's trust.

Living With Awareness and Lightness

Awareness means noticing without judging.

You notice:

When you need rest

When you're pushing too hard

When stress is accumulating

When joy is available

Lightness comes from responding early instead of waiting until burnout forces you to stop.

This is the quiet mastery you've been building all along.

Conclusion — A New Rhythm of Living

This was never just a detox.

It was a return.

A return to listening instead of forcing.

To nourishing instead of restricting.

To living in rhythm instead of reaction.

You didn't remove stress from your life—you changed your relationship with it.

You learned how to:

- Calm your body
- Feed your nervous system
- Respect your energy
- Trust your signals
- Recover without fear

And most importantly, you learned that peace is not

something you earn after everything is done.

It's something you practice—daily, imperfectly, gently.

There will still be busy days. Emotional seasons. Unexpected challenges.

But now, stress no longer defines you.

You have a rhythm to return to.

A body you trust.

A calm you can access.

This is not the end of a program.

It's the beginning of a new way of living—where nourishment replaces urgency, awareness replaces overwhelm, and joy becomes daily medicine.

You are not behind.

You are not broken.

You are already on your way.

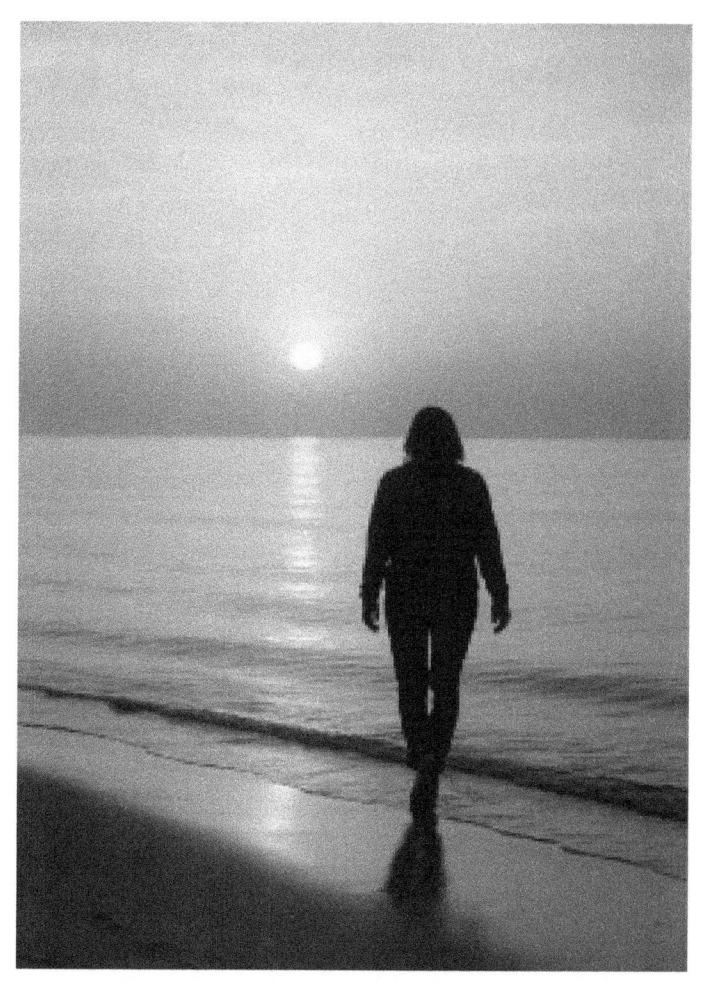

Acknowledgment

I wish to thank the countless individuals—readers, health practitioners, and nutrition experts—who have inspired this work. Your questions, insights, and shared experiences shaped this book into something practical and accessible. Above all, I am grateful to the community of everyday people seeking healthier, more energized lives; your determination proves that transformation is always possible.

www.ingramcontent.com/pod-product-compliance
Lightning Source LLC
Chambersburg PA
CBHW050841040426
42333CB00058B/227